The Easy Guide
To Understanding and Managing Your Asthma

Table of Contents

Introduction

Ignorance about the disease of asthma kills. Knowledge about asthma saves lives. This book will teach you how to recognize the signs of asthma. How to correctly identify the asthma severity category based on symptoms, pulmonary function, interference with your daily activities, or your use of quick-relief medicines. This book will answer questions you need to know the answers to like; Do I have asthma? How do I know when and how to use my medicine? How do I use the different devices the asthma medicines come with? What is a peak flow meter and why do I need one? Will I grow out of this? Can I still engage in my favorite sport? How does my medicine work? What's happening inside my lungs when I'm having an asthma attack?

First we'll discuss exactly what asthma is and why it's dangerous. Various definitions of asthma have been used over the years but as the medical community has learned more about the disease, the definition has been made more and more accurate. In this book we'll explain how your various asthma medicines work by pointing to it's place of action within the current asthma definition. We'll discuss at length how the various asthma devices are used and point out the things you should always do and the things that you should never do. We'll explain what a trigger is and how to avoid them. We'll make this often complicated subject of asthma a simple matter that you'll easily be able to understand and remember.

In *The Easy Guide to Understanding and Managing Your Asthma*, you'll find charts and forms which will guide you in treating, measuring the severity of, and managing your asthma. Virtually all of this information can be found in the Expert Panel's third report on asthma but that body of work was written by professionals for professionals. This book has been written for you or any non-medical person. Simple principles about understanding how to recognize and manage your asthma.

As each topic is explained, we'll move seamlessly into the next, with the overall goal of making you fully understand just what you're dealing with in asthma. What it is, how to treat it, what your medicines are all about and how they fit into the management of asthma, how to use the different asthma devices and many other concerns which other books on asthma fail to mention.

The Easy Guide to Understanding and Managing Your Asthma will leave you with a deeper understanding on just what asthma is and how your effective management of it will help you to retake control of your life.

The Expert Panel

Throughout this book you'll hear a lot about the Expert Panel and what the Panel recommends. Just who is this 'Expert Panel'?

The coordinating committee of the National Asthma Education and Prevention Program recommended that the guidelines for treating and managing asthma be reviewed. Many steps were taken to make sure that the guidelines were based on research and the best practices of 'experts' in the management and treatment of asthma. The guidelines were then given to a panel of guidelines endusers who were to give feedback about the guidelines. Finally a copy of the guidelines were posted on the website of the National Heart, Lung, and Blood Institute so the public could see it and comment on it before the guidelines for asthma management would be finalized and released.

The Third Expert Panel on the diagnosis and management of asthma are listed by their name, the organization and medical or research facility they are or were associated with at the time they were asked to participate, and its location.

William W. Busse, M.D., Chair
University of Wisconsin Medical School
Madison, Wisconsin

Homer A. Boushey, M.D.
University of California–San Francisco
San Francisco, California

Carlos A. Camargo, Jr., M.D., Dr.P.H.
Massachusetts General Hospital
Boston, Massachusetts

David Evans, Ph.D., A.E.-C,
Columbia University
New York, New York

Michael B. Foggs, M.D.
Advocate Health Centers
Chicago, Illinois

Susan L. Janson, D.N.Sc., R.N., A.N.P.,
F.A.A.N.
University of California–San Francisco
San Francisco, California

H. William Kelly, Pharm.D.
University of New Mexico Health Sciences Center
Albuquerque, New Mexico

Robert F. Lemanske, M.D.
University of Wisconsin Hospital and Clinics
Madison, Wisconsin

Fernando D. Martinez, M.D.
University of Arizona Medical Center
Tucson, Arizona

Robert J. Meyer, M.D.
U.S. Food and Drug Administration
Silver Spring, Maryland

Harold S. Nelson, M.D.
National Jewish Medical and Research Center
Denver, Colorado

Thomas A. E. Platts-Mills, M.D., Ph.D.
University of Virginia School of Medicine
Charlottesville, Virginia

Michael Schatz, M.D., M.S.
Kaiser-Permanente–San Diego
San Diego, California

Gail Shapiro, M.D.
University of Washington
Seattle, Washington

Stuart Stoloff, M.D.
University of Nevada School of Medicine
Carson City, Nevada

Stanley J. Szefler, M.D.
National Jewish Medical and Research Center
Denver, Colorado

Scott T. Weiss, M.D., M.S.
Brigham and Women's Hospital
Boston, Massachusetts

Barbara P. Yawn, M.D., M.Sc.
Olmstead Medical Center
Rochester, Minnesota

What is Asthma?

Most books on asthma use a different definition for asthma. In 2007 the Expert Panel (a panel of asthma researchers, teachers, and clinicians) produced its third report and in that report gave one of the best definitions for asthma:

Asthma is a chronic inflammatory disorder of the airways in which many cells and cellular elements play a role: in particular, mast cells, eosinophils, neutrophils (especially in sudden onset, fatal exacerbations, occupational asthma, and patients who smoke), T lymphocytes, macrophages, and epithelial cells. In susceptible individuals, this inflammation causes recurrent episodes of coughing (particularly at night or early in the morning), wheezing, breathlessness, and chest tightness. These episodes are usually associated with widespread but variable airflow obstruction that is often reversible either spontaneously or with treatment.

This is probably the most complete definition of asthma. It mentions one of the core difficulties with asthma as part of what defines asthma--inflammation. This definition points out several of the cell types thought to be closely involved in asthma attacks, or flare-ups. Then those symptoms with which every asthmatic has had to deal at one time or another are mentioned. This definition is very accurate and most useful but you might still be grasping for understanding. What exactly **is** asthma? If I have it how did I get it? Is it contagious? Was I born with it?

The medical community have learned quite a bit about asthma but it is still not completely understood. We believe that it can be inherited. If your parents had it, particularly your mother, there is a good chance that you could have it too. There is a genetic component to asthma but it is still not possible to predict with certainty who will or will not be born with it.

Asthma isn't contagious. If your significant other has asthma, it doesn't matter if you hug and kiss them daily, you won't get asthma that way. Fortunately, it isn't sexually transmitted either. Even if an asthmatic coughs directly in your face daily (heaven forbid), you would still not contract asthma.

There are a couple of theories on how you could *develop* asthma. It is believed that if you are exposed to certain environmental allergens at a young enough age, asthma could develop. That is, the symptoms of asthma such as wheezing, coughing, and/or hypersensitive airways could start becoming a problem. Allergens such as dust mites or molds are often the reason the airways become extra sensitive (hypersensitive). If the child contracts a respiratory virus, namely the respiratory syncytial virus (known as RSV), an asthma-like condition could develop.

It isn't always the very young who can suddenly 'get' asthma. Sometimes grownups can find themselves dealing with symptoms of shortness of breath, wheezing, and nighttime coughing and for all practical purposes these adults have contracted asthma. In cases like these, we would refer to their condition as *occupational* asthma since it is likely that the condition developed as a result of exposure to some allergen or irritant to which the person came in contact at work. If you work in an environment where there is exposure to dust or some type of air-borne chemical and if you are vulnerable, asthma could develop.

Now the question arises 'well who is vulnerable?'

There is a theory referred to as Innate Immunity. This idea suggests that if a person is exposed to many of these allergens while they are young, they will be less likely to develop asthma because their immune system will have built effective defenses against it. They would be less susceptible to the development of asthma. For example, if you are born and raised in a rural environment with several brothers and sisters, you would be less likely to develop asthma. Early exposure to airway irritants and allergens would help prepare the airway against extra sensitivity. Older siblings would share their viruses in the simple course of living and the unfiltered outdoors air would together help build up the airway defenses. In this scenario you would expect that the diet would be more wholesome and this has some positive bearing on the resistance to the development of asthma.

These are only theories but more is becoming understood about how you might come to have asthma. Someday it might be possible to predict who will and who won't develop asthma before a single symptom is experienced.

The Abnormal Asthma Airway

Pathophysiology is the medical term to describe tissue behavior when it's abnormal. Patho- is a prefix suggesting abnormality or illness and physiology pertains to function. So asthma pathophysiology is in effect an asthmatic's lung tissue function. Another way of seeing pathophysiology is by asking what's going on in the lungs of an asthmatic. To help you to understand this, let's look at the definition of asthma again.

Asthma is a chronic inflammatory disorder of the airways in which many cells and cellular elements play a role: in particular, mast cells, eosinophils, neutrophils (especially in sudden onset, fatal exacerbations, occupational asthma, and patients who smoke), T lymphocytes, macrophages, and epithelial cells. In susceptible individuals, this inflammation causes recurrent episodes of coughing (particularly at night or early in the morning), wheezing, breathlessness, and chest tightness. These episodes are usually associated with widespread but variable airflow obstruction that is often reversible either spontaneously or with treatment.

Inflammation is at the heart of the problem in asthma. What is inflammation? When tissue is injured, it seeks to protect itself from what has injured it. Swelling, seepage of fluids from vessels in the area of the injury, and general loss of function are consequences of this process. More vessels grow and mucus secretions increase. Over time, the original design of the airway is changed for the worse and the airway becomes much less efficient as a passageway for air movement.

You experience this swollen airway with more secretions in it as difficulty breathing and chest tightness. As the air struggles to push it's way along a smaller air passageway due to swelling and increased secretions, wheezing is heard. Wheezing is a high pitched noise caused by the movement of air through tight air passageways. Sometimes the airways can get so tight as a result of swelling and overreaction to allergens that there is virtually no movement of air at all.

How and why does all this lung damage happen? First, you have to be vulnerable to it. Whether you've been lucky enough to inherit it from your family, develop it as a result of early lung injury from disease or typically, from something in the air, your lungs are now hypersensitive and are inclined to overreact to many different things. This explanation is not meant to be perfectly complete in listing all the ways you can become 'asthmatic' but simply tries to show how this problem develops and how it behaves going forward.

We now have a vulnerable pair of lungs, we'll call him Joe Asthmatic. Joe does well most of the time. He can engage in normal physical activities. He seldom has problems breathing unless he's exposed to dust mites. Dust mites are little microscopic bugs that live in house dust and usually inhabit beds and pillows. So Joe is sleeping on his pillow and breathes in some dust mites. In the individual with non-asthmatic lungs, these dust mites will attract macrophages who will round them up and throw them out. Think of a bouncer in a club. Macrophages are large cells whose job is to 'bounce' any unwanted thing that comes into the lung. In an asthmatic lung, the bouncer overreacts and calls the police who then alerts the National Guard. All these heavily armed men destroys the club in their enthusiasm to aid the bouncer.

This analogy is used to avoid the technical discussion of long cellular names and processes to describe just what happens when the body's immune system overreacts to allergens. The key point here is 'overreaction.' This cellular overreaction is the culprit which ultimately narrows the airways and causes Joe Asthmatic so much breathing trouble.

Categories of Asthma

Asthma attacks can range from appearing infrequently to occurring virtually all the time. The EPR-3 has divided this range of severity into four categories based on how often you need quick-relief medicine, how often you have symptoms of breathing trouble, how often your sleep is interrupted by nighttime episodes of troubled breathing, by how much your asthma condition interferes with your normal daily activity, and any measurable change in your lung function. Based on these criteria for dividing asthma into categories of severity, the Expert Panel has given us four categories. Let's discuss each of them in turn.

Note: *In the interest of better understanding the categories of asthma severity as it pertains to lung function, let's quickly talk about Forced Expired Volume and Peak Flows.*

Since asthma is a disease that makes it difficult to breathe air out of the lungs, some tests have been developed to measure how hard it is to breathe air out. Probably the most important test is called the Forced Expired Volume. The time it takes for an asthmatic to blow out or forcefully expire a deep breath is a telling measure of asthma severity. The longer it takes to breathe out, the worse the asthma condition. This expired volume is measured using several different increments of time but the measurement over 1 second is most useful for appreciating the differences between the asthma categories.

Peak flow is also a test to gauge how hard it is to blow air out. Instead of measuring the volume over time, a peak flow meter simply measures the volume. The smaller a volume is that can be quickly blown out of the lungs, the more severe the asthma condition has become. These tests provide some objective help to a person with asthma in understanding how bad is his or her condition.

Intermittent

Intermittent is the least severe category. Let's suppose that Joe Asthmatic is in the 'intermittent' category of asthma severity. Joe has his quick-relief inhaler just in case he starts having breathing trouble. Fortunately, he seldom needs it. In fact, he needed it only twice last week. His asthma condition is well controlled and gives him very little trouble. In all of last month he awoke only two times at night as a direct result of problems with his asthma. When at work he doesn't think twice about whether he should take the elevator or the stairs. On the weekends he indulges himself in playful sports competitions with his friends with no problems. Generally, forced expired volumes aren't done on a daily or weekly basis in the home. One has to go to a doctor's office or pulmonary function lab for this test. Peak flow meters can be personally owned and is very helpful in keeping asthmatics aware of their lungs condition. Joe performs his peak flow every few days but it's virtually always within 80% of what is normal for Joe. Only once in this entire year has Joe required an oral corticosteroid to regain control of his asthma. You might say that Joe Asthmatic is happily living his life with few reminders that he even has asthma.

Mild Persistent

The next to the least severe is the Mild Persistent category. Now, let's suppose that Joe is in this category. Joe is mindful to keep up with his quick-relief inhaler. He has found that he needs it on average more than twice weekly. Fortunately for Joe he very rarely needs it more that once on the day he does use it. At night his sleep is sometimes interrupted by his asthma difficulties. Between three and four times a month he awakes with shortness of breath or chest tightness. When he's at work he does have to give a little thought to whether he should take the stairs or ride the elevator. It does matter to Joe since on a bad day for him, taking the stairs might not be advisable since his symptoms usually bother him more than two or three times weekly. However, he doesn't have to deal with breathing symptoms on a daily basis. Recently, he had pulmonary functions performed and was glad to find that he was within 80% of what is normal for himself and for others of his height and gender. The pulmonary functions were recommended after he required a second prescription for oral steroids this year despite his consistent daily use of a low dose inhaled corticosteroid. Overall Joe manages his asthma condition well.

Moderate Persistent

Moderate Persistent asthma is next to the most severe category. Let's consider what it would be like for Joe if he were categorized as Moderate Persistent. Joe knows the importance of keeping his prescriptions for his quick-relief medicine filled since he uses it every day. Not a day goes by that he doesn't feel some level of breathing distress. Some days it's chest tightness or excessive coughing. On other days it might be a simple inability to get a deep breath. In any case, he needs his quick-relief medicine to help him deal with his asthma. Nighttime awakenings marked by breathing troubles can be counted on to occur at least once a week but most often more than once a week. It doesn't happen every night but it happens all too often for Joe. His condition definitely causes some limitations when it comes to his daily life. He never takes the stairs because he could provoke an attack by doing so. For Joe, if the elevator is slow, he'll just have to wait. His pulmonary function tests say that his lungs are functioning within a range above 60% of where it should be but considerably below 80%. He consistently takes his longterm control medicines: A low dose inhaled corticosteroid along with a long acting beta agonist (these medicines will be discussed in detail in a later chapter). Despite his consistent attention to his longterm medicines, he has still required three prescriptions for oral corticosteroids during this year. Joe must be constantly watchful of his asthma to maintain control and avoid hospitalization.

Severe Persistent

Now let's consider how it is for Joe when dealing with the most severe category of the four asthma categories. Joe has severe persistent asthma. He uses his quick-relief medicine several times a day since his symptoms never stop. You can always see his breathing distress reflected in his face as he goes about his day. His breathing troubles wake him virtually every night as a result of coughing excessively, wheezing, chest tightness or something else. He dutifully takes his longterm medicines of medium dose corticosteroids and long acting beta agonists and his doctors are considering raising his dose. Joe is barely able to work and is looking into relocating to a drier climate. He has become a regular at the local emergency department and has been hospitalized more than once. Each time he's been in the hospital he has had to take oral steroids. His lungs are functioning below 60% of what they should be based on his age and height. Joe needs to follow his doctors advice in every detail and do all that he can to prevent a deterioration of his condition. This includes monitoring his environment so that he controls the triggers he can control and avoid those triggers he can't control.

The Expert Panel's third report created these four categories of asthma which are separated by the frequency of symptoms, use of quick-relief medicines, limitations on daily activity, frequency of nighttime awakenings, and lung function.

Joe Asthmatic is a young adult in these scenarios. The same criteria are used for children too but there are a few slight differences when determining where one category ends and another begins. Tables defining asthma categories for the different age groups can be found in the additional resources section.

Understanding Pulmonary Functions

What is pulmonary function testing? You might have heard your doctor mention pulmonary function testing when discussing your asthma. It could just as easily be called Lung Testing but pulmonary is the medical term used when referring to the lung.

Pulmonary function testing or sometimes just called pulmonary functions, includes many types of tests designed to measure the level of function of the lungs. Some pulmonary function tests measure lung volumes. Some tests measure how quickly the lungs can be emptied of air. Other tests measure how effective the lung is at taking in oxygen and disposing of carbon dioxide. There are a large number of different pulmonary function tests and each test is selected to yield specific information.

Certain tests are very helpful in separating one lung disease from another. Consider the Law School Admissions Test (LSAT). This test is given to applicants to separate candidates who would possibly make good lawyers from those who possibly wouldn't make good lawyers. The Medical College Admissions Test (MCAT) provides the same separating function for those who would possibly make good doctors. There are pulmonary function tests which can help a clinician separate one lung disease from another. What the pulmonary test really does is uncover certain lung 'behavior' which is more likely to be one disease than another. Pulmonary function tests are also performed just to show how well the lung is working. Let's consider a few pulmonary function tests and how they might be helpful.

Forced Expired Volume tests measure how fast a person can blow air out of the lungs. This test can help separate lungs which can be emptied of air quickly from lungs which takes a little more time. Asthmatic lungs are well known to be unable to empty quickly. Generally, an asthma patient has an easier time breathing air in than breathing air out. A forced expired volume test would measure what is a normal amount of time for most of the air to be out against the time it took the air to actually get out. This test is useful when testing for asthma since slower than normal expired volumes are normal for asthma.

Lung Capacity tests measures how much air is in the lung.

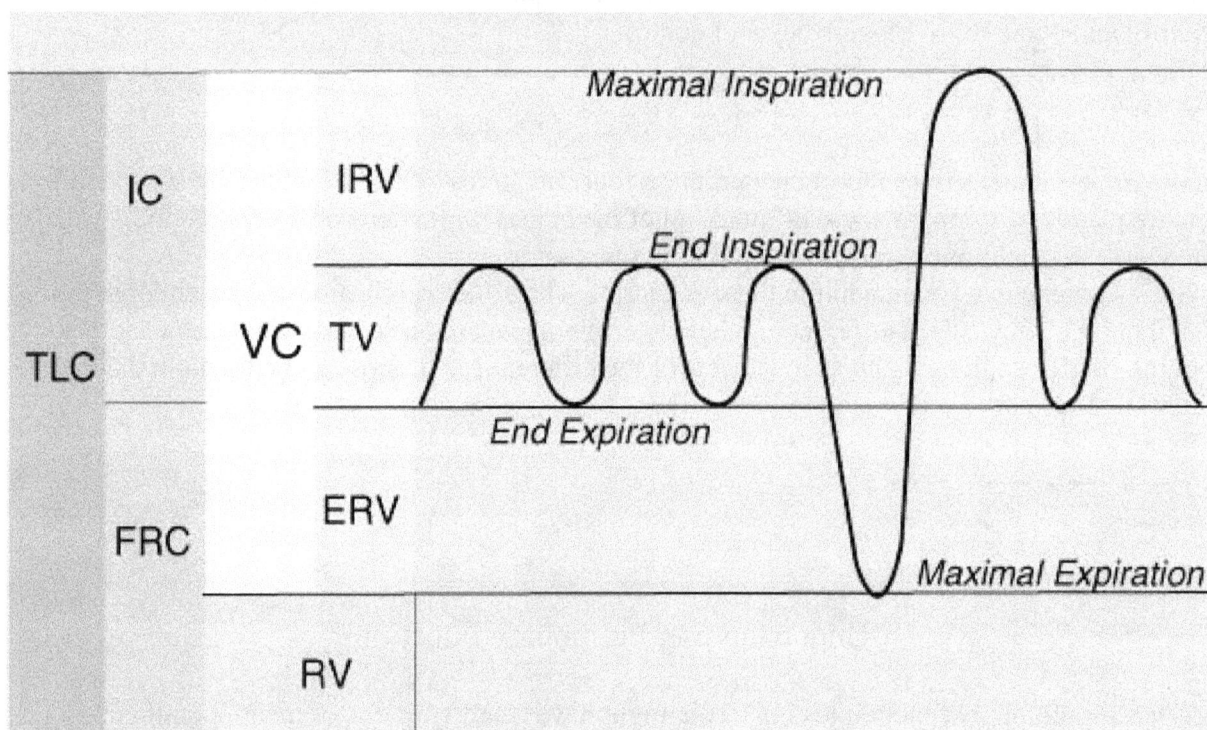

Tests which measure capacity would be useful to separate diseases which limit how much air a lung can take in from diseases that don't effect the lung in that way. An example would be the disease Sarcoidosis. This disease happens to limit how much air a lung can hold. A test which measures lung capacity wouldn't tell the clinician specifically that this disease **is** Sarcoidosis but it would help narrow the list of diseases that it could be.

The Flow Volume Loop is another test which can be very useful to both tell how well a lung is functioning and to help separate certain diseases from other diseases.

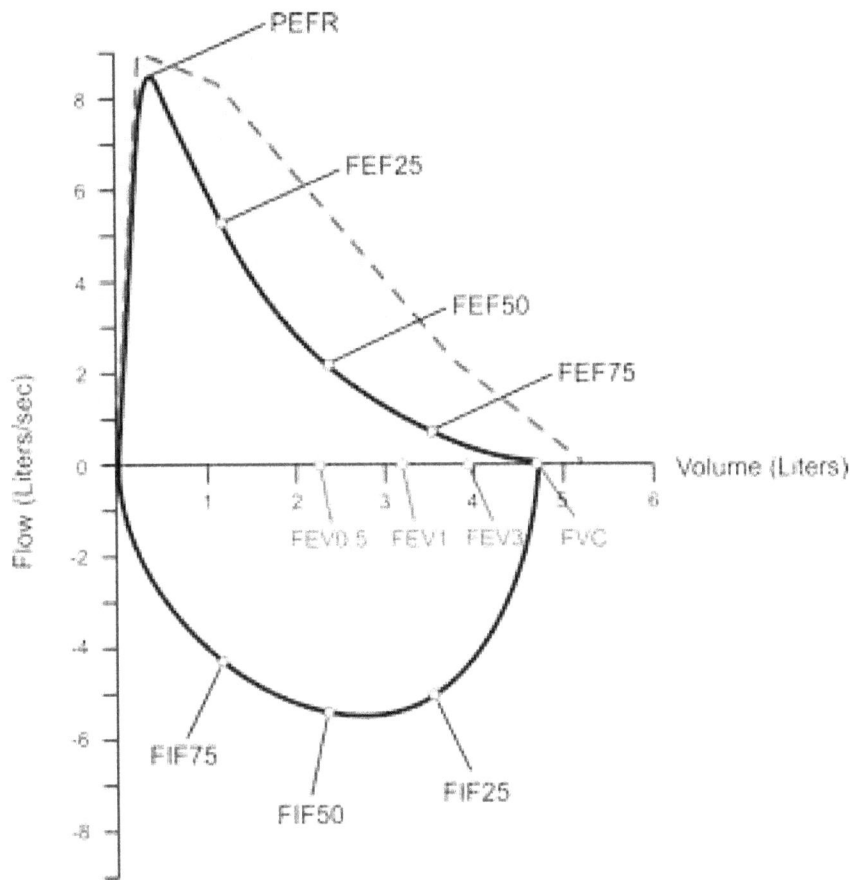

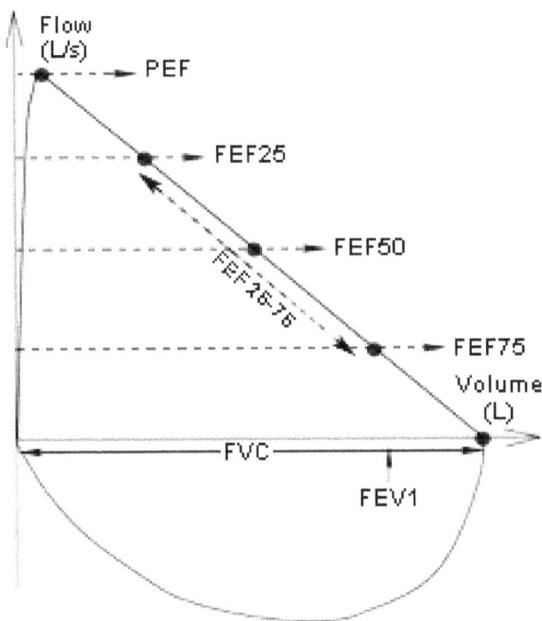

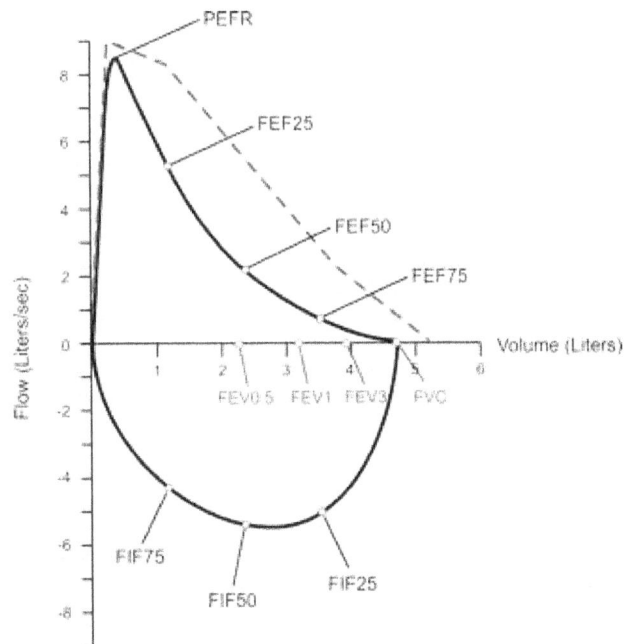

This test is performed by measuring all the air that is breathed out completely then sucked back in completely. A computer draws a picture which represents the air as it is blown out and sucked back in. The shape of that picture can tell many useful things to the clinician. Certain diseases make certain shapes of pictures during this flow volume loop test and this information can help narrow the list of possible diseases. This test can also help determine the improving health or failing health of a particular set of lungs by comparing a past test with a current test.

There are many different pulmonary function tests and each of them has a particular best use. This short discussion of pulmonary functions is not expected to show you the relevance of every test. Understanding how lung testing can inform a clinician of the lungs' condition is important to recognizing how some tests can make your asthma easier to manage. The Expert Panel recommends that asthmatics should have pulmonary function tests performed every year or two but especially if there has been a serious flare-up. Tests which are most useful in the diagnosis or management of asthma will be explained as they come up in our discussion.

Distinguishing Asthma From Other Conditions

Asthma is an obstructive pulmonary disease. When you have asthma, particularly during a period when there is difficulty breathing, air is hard to expel. That's where the word 'obstructive' comes in when describing asthma. An asthmatic is less able to rapidly blow air out than a non-asthmatic. A pulmonary function test which measures how fast air can be expelled from the lungs would be useful in telling asthma from other diseases.

Another important sign that you're dealing with asthma is its reversibility or partial reversibility of the breathing difficulty. Air flow obstruction is being reversed when you get some relief after taking your quick-relief medicine. Reversibility of the air flow obstruction either by itself or after using a short acting beta agonist is a characteristic of asthma.

Family history of asthma, frequent recurring wheezing, worsening symptoms during or just after exercise or sensitivity to certain inhaled allergens are additional signs that asthma is the likely disease. There are other signs which point to asthma but let's consider some other diseases or conditions which might at first glance appear to be asthma.

Bronchiolitis

Bronchiolitis causes little children to have trouble breathing. You'll hear wheezing and you'll see the classic signs of trouble breathing like flaring of the nose, fast breathing and tugging of the windpipe (called tracheal tugging). These signs would also be present in asthma. How do you tell the difference?

The medicines used to treat asthma are also sometimes used to treat bronchiolitis (often called by the name of the virus most commonly associated with it, RSV). Quick-relief medicines like albuterol or levalbuterol are sometimes used and are occasionally helpful. Most of the time these bronchodilators don't help if you're dealing with bronchiolitis.

Bronchiolitis or RSV(Respiratory Syncytial Virus) has an easily identifiable signature. Bronchiolitis usually happens during the late fall and winter months. Asthma can happen during any month. Small children are usually the ones effected by bronchiolitis while asthma will effect anyone of any age. Bronchiolitis typically follows a cold or appears to be the worsening of a cold. You'll see lot's of nasal secretions with bronchiolitis and often all you can do to help is keep the nasal passages open by bulb suctioning.

Of course, if your little one is having trouble breathing you should take him or her to a doctor and allow the child to be professionally evaluated. With the review of medical history and a physical examination, your doctor can likely determine what the true issue is and treat it.

Croup

  Like bronchiolitis, croup is also caused by a virus. Croup is also known by the extremely long and hard to pronounce name of laryngotracheobronchitis. This long name identifies the location of the viral infection. It's in the throat in the area where the voice box is found. The child's cough is usually described as a seal-like bark which is explained by the location of the infection.
  Croup usually effects small children between the ages of six months and five or six years old. It can be occasionally found in children as old as eleven or twelve but this isn't common. Teenagers are almost never seen with croup.
  The image below is that of an x-ray of a child's neck. Notice the area between the arrows. This is where there is swelling and it is this narrowing of the airway that causes the barking cough and the high pitched breathing noise.

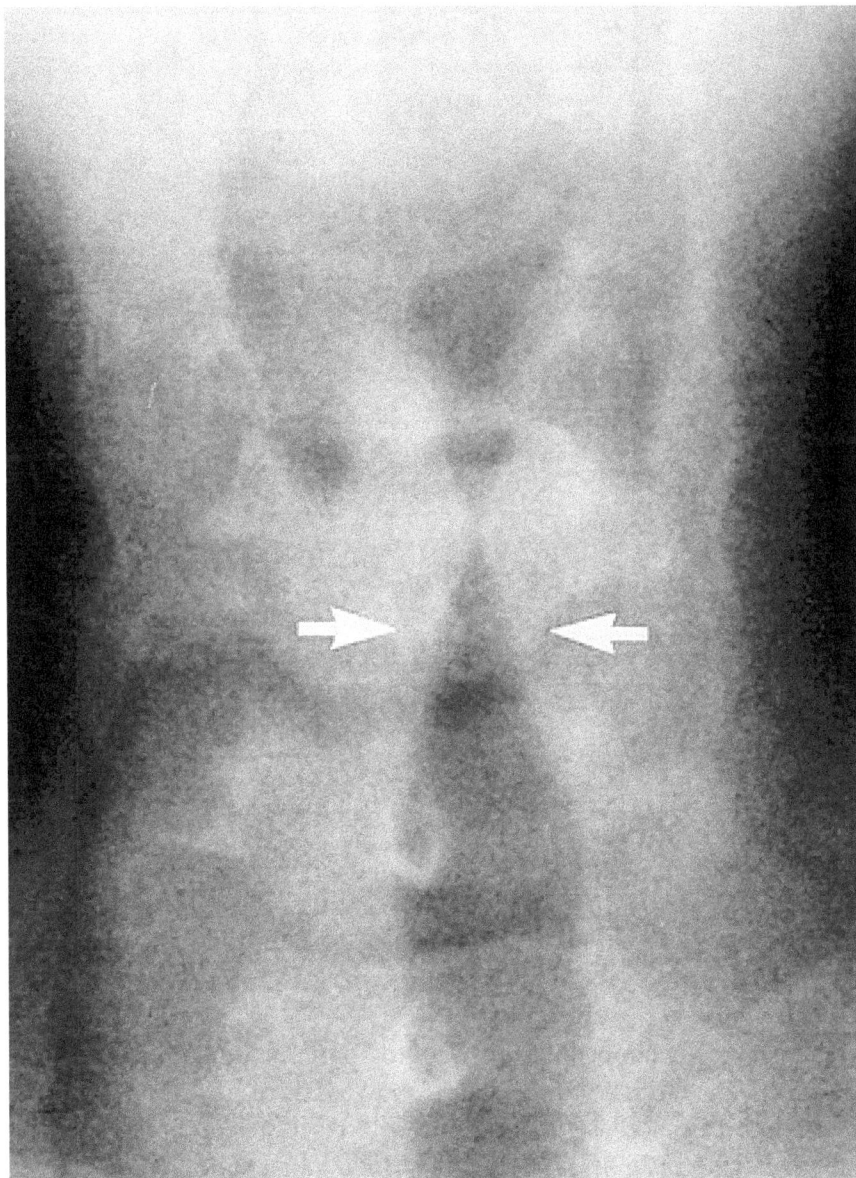

Quick-relief medicines do little to help with the symptoms of croup. In the event your child has the classic barking cough, high pitched breathing noise, or husky voice, you should take the child to an emergency department right away. Croup isn't often fatal but it could be something else causing the symptoms. A foreign body caught in the airway or a bacterial infection of the lid to the windpipe (called the glottis) could be the real problem. X-rays and professional assessment could determine what the problem really is with your child.

Foreign Bodies

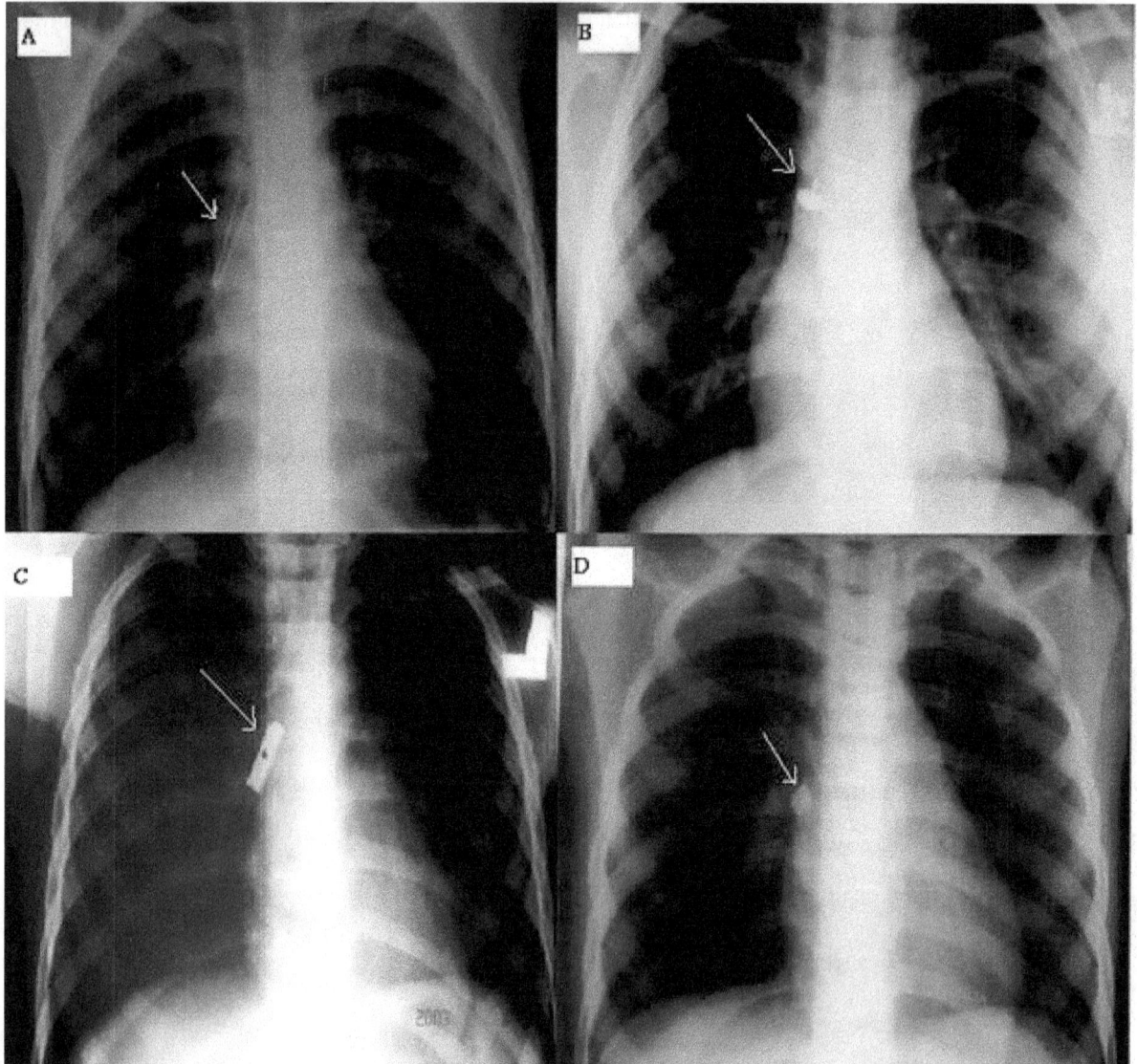

Particularly in children, something like a bead, peanut, or small toy part could be inhaled into the lung and lodge itself in an airway. The child would possibly show signs of breathing difficulty and wheezing. There might be an increase in coughing with periodic attempts to dislodge the object. There might even be a drop of oxygen in the blood (if taken to doctor's office or ER where an oxygen saturation could be taken).

Initially this problem might appear to be asthma since asthma often presents itself in much the same way. However, if given a short acting beta agonist, there will likely be little or no relief. Some history review might reveal that the child is inclined to put things into his or her mouth or that the family has no history of asthma or that this is the very first sign of these symptoms. Asthma would probably have shown itself before now.

The treatment of symptoms resulting from a foreign body always revolve around the removal of that item from the airway.

Vocal Cord Dysfunction

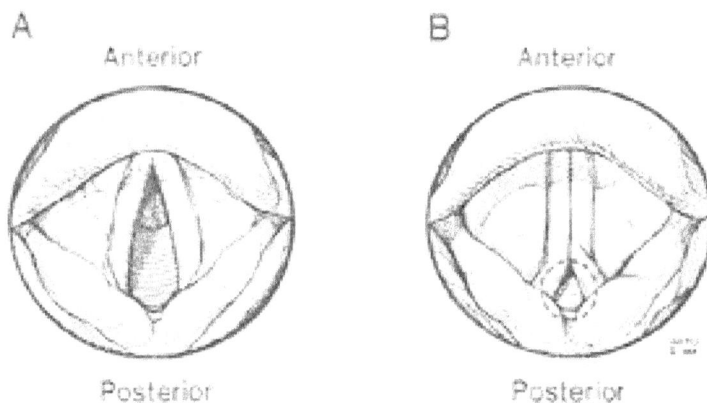

What is vocal cord dysfunction? The American Thoracic Society's Patient Information Series discusses this condition at http://www.patients.thoracic.org. The important things to know about VCD (Vocal Cord Dysfunction) is that it presents itself in much the same way as asthma. If you're experiencing VCD you might feel breathless, have throat or chest tightness, you could possibly be wheezing or have some other form of noisy breathing. VCD can also be started up by some of the same things that can start an asthma attack: respiratory viruses, smoke, strong emotions or exercise. The one sure way to tell asthma and VCD apart is to have a doctor look into the throat while the dysfunction is taking place.

VCD is when the vocal cords don't function normally. Normally the cords open when you breath in and out as in figure A. When there is vocal cord 'dysfunction,' the cords close when they should be opening as in figure B. Quick-Relief medicines won't help this condition. If VCD can be definitely diagnosed, the cause of it must be treated. If it's stress or overexcitement that starts it up, you'll have to learn to control your emotions better. If it's gastroesophageal reflux disease (GERD) that's causing the problem, your doctor will help you find treatment for that. If it's exercise in cold weather that's causing VCD, you'll have to cover your mouth and nose with a scarf when you exercise outdoors or you'll have to exercise indoors.

The main treatment for VCD itself is speech therapy. A therapist experienced in the treatment of Vocal Cord Dysfunction will be able to teach you how to relax your throat muscles and in this way cause your vocal cords to regain normal function.

Tracheal Stenosis

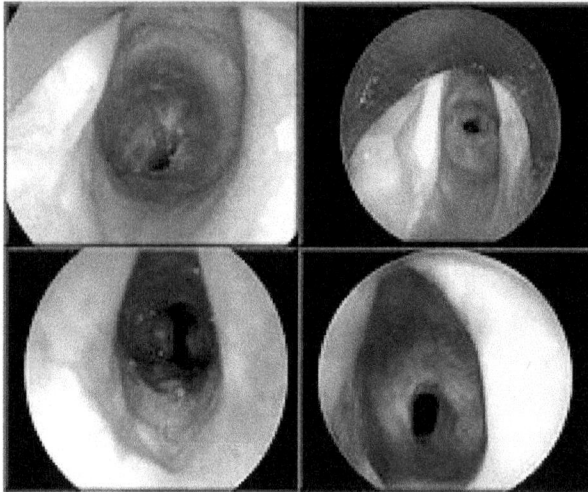

Tracheal stenosis can negatively effect breathing and lead some to suspect asthma as the culprit. The above images is what the windpipe with stenosis looks like if you were looking at it from inside your throat. Stenosis means 'narrowing.' The breathing hole is smaller than it should be.

If you're experiencing difficult breathing or shortness of breath while you're doing light activities, this sounds similar to what you might experience with asthma. However, tracheal stenosis slows down air coming in and asthma airways slows air going out.

Tracheal stenosis is the narrowing of a section of the trachea or windpipe. This narrowing can be high or low on the windpipe. It usually occurs higher up in the windpipe in children than in adults. This could be caused by a respiratory virus, scarring from previous endotracheal intubation (a tube inserted into your windpipe to have a machine breath for you), or damage from stomach acids seeping into the esophagus (GERD). There are other possible causes but the important thing to know is that quick-relief medicines prescribed for asthma will not help. Doctors can find out what it is by getting an upper airway x-ray or bronchoscopy (which involves looking through the nose or mouth into the upper throat to see the narrowing).

Allergic Rhinitis and Sinusitis

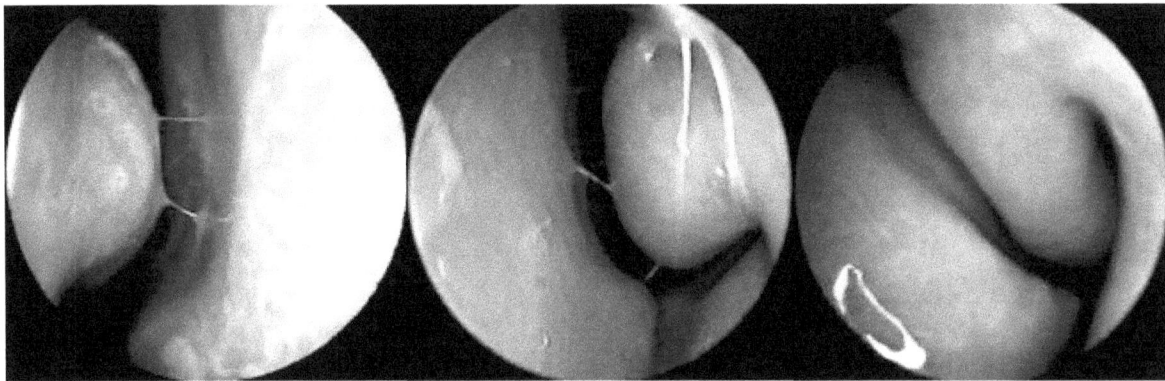

Allergic rhinitis is associated with the itching and sneezing that you do when something in the air is irritating your nose. Sinusitis is the infection of your sinuses. Neither of these conditions are generally mistaken for asthma but both contribute to the ease or difficulty of treating asthma.

The medical community agrees that asthma can be better controlled if rhinitis and sinusitis are treated when they're present. In other words, your asthma can't be treated while your rhinitis is ignored if your asthma is to be controlled.

Treatment of excessive nasal itching, runny nose and sneezing can be effectively treated with a nasal steroid spray. The image below is an example of a nasal steroid spray.

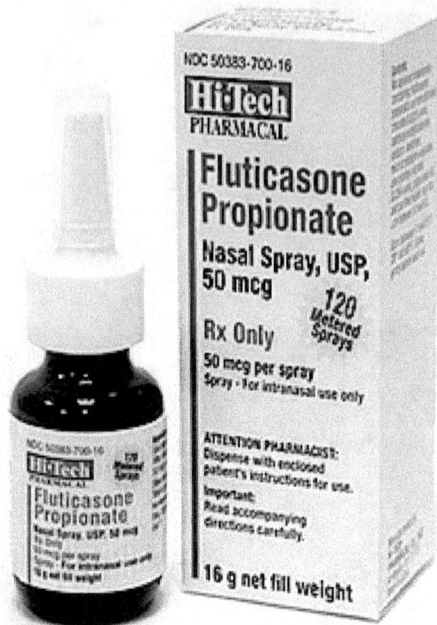

Oral antihistamines have also been used to effectively control flareups of rhinitis. The point which should not be missed here is that rhinitis and sinusitis can cause your asthma to be hard to control. These conditions should be managed along with your asthma.

Gastroesophageal Reflux Disease

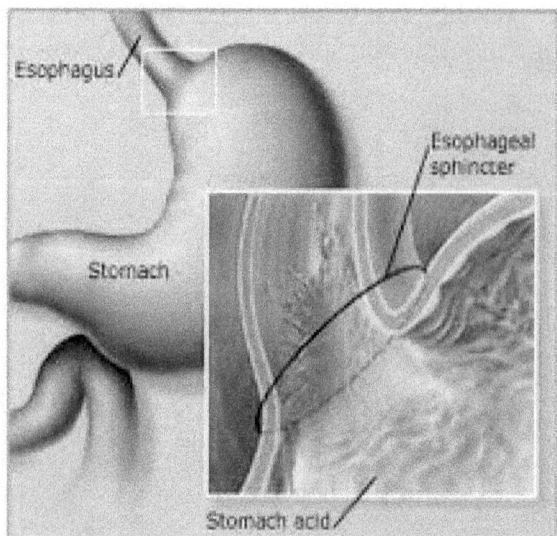

Gastroesophageal reflux disease, referred to as GERD for short, can be mistaken for asthma at first glance. Symptoms such as nighttime awakenings due to difficulty breathing and wheezing will immediately bring asthma to the clinicians mind. This tendency for GERD to be confused with asthma certainly can complicate the diagnosis of asthma.

Gastroesophageal reflux is caused by the seepage of gastric contents back up and into the esophagus. The esophagus is the passageway connecting the mouth and the stomach. Food and water should travel only one way--from the mouth to the stomach. When stomach contents which are saturated with gastric acids seeps back into the esophagus, these substances can find their way onto the vocal cords causing hoarse voice and into the lungs causing wheezing. When you lay down to sleep, the seepage of the contents occur even easier and you might awake with chest discomfort and breathing difficulty.

Treatment of GERD revolves around eating smaller meals, eating several hours before laying down, sleeping at an upwardly inclined angle, and avoiding foods which tend to make more acid. Sometimes medicines are used to help limit the amount of acid your stomach produces.

If you think that you might have gastroesophageal reflux, talk with your doctor for help with diagnosis and treatment.

Heart Disease

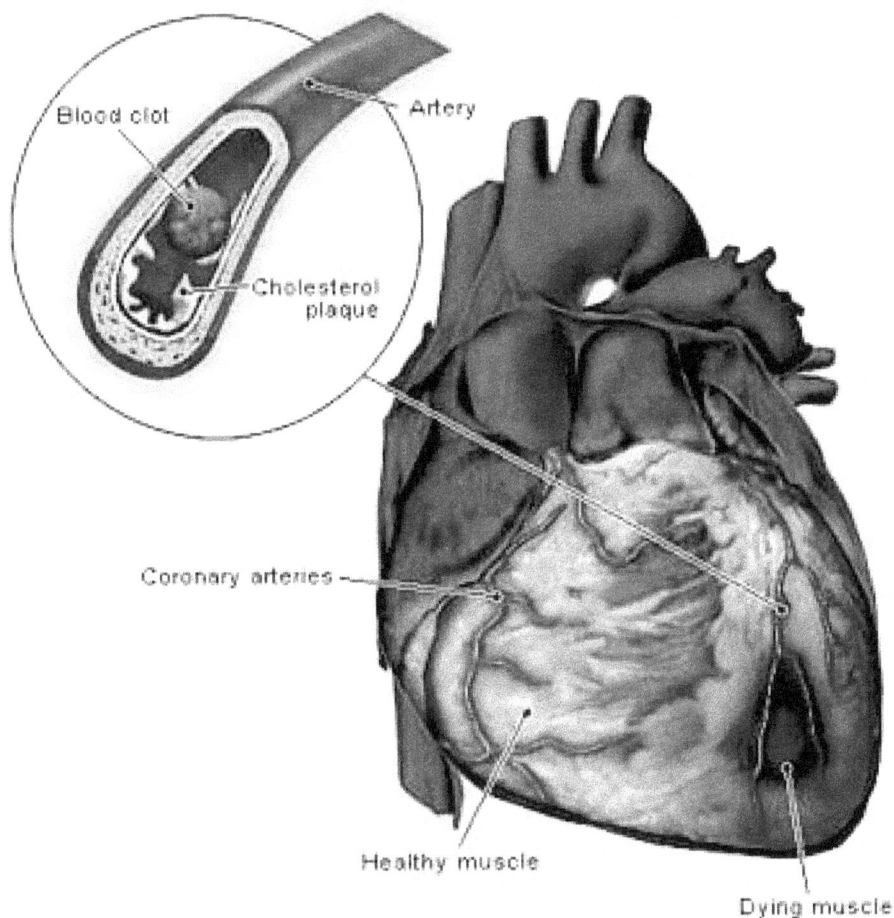

No age group is absolutely immune from heart disease but adults tend to have to deal with this condition more often than children. If you're unsure whether it is heart disease or asthma that is causing you to wake up with chest tightness and difficulty breathing, consider this: Do your legs swell? If they do, it is probably not asthma you're dealing with but heart disease. Do quick-relief inhalers like albuterol give you relief from your breathing difficulty? If they do, it's probably not heart disease giving you the trouble but asthma. Are your neck veins distended (puffed up)? If they are, asthma is probably not your problem. Have you ever felt better after using nitroglycerin? Nitroglycerin can help some heart problems but it never helps an asthma flare-up. Of course you could be dealing with both asthma and heart disease combined. You should always let your doctor evaluate you to help you understand what you can do to improve your overall health. This book might be useful in helping you to understand some of what you might be dealing with but you will always need your doctor's involvement to be sure.

Obesity

Obesity could cause a number of the same complaints as asthma. Shortness of breath after just a little exercise. Difficulty getting a good nights sleep due to waking up at night with trouble breathing. Even wheezing might be heard during heavy exertion.

There are several levels of obesity. This image isn't meant to perfectly match the levels of obesity but is intended to show what increasing obesity looks like.

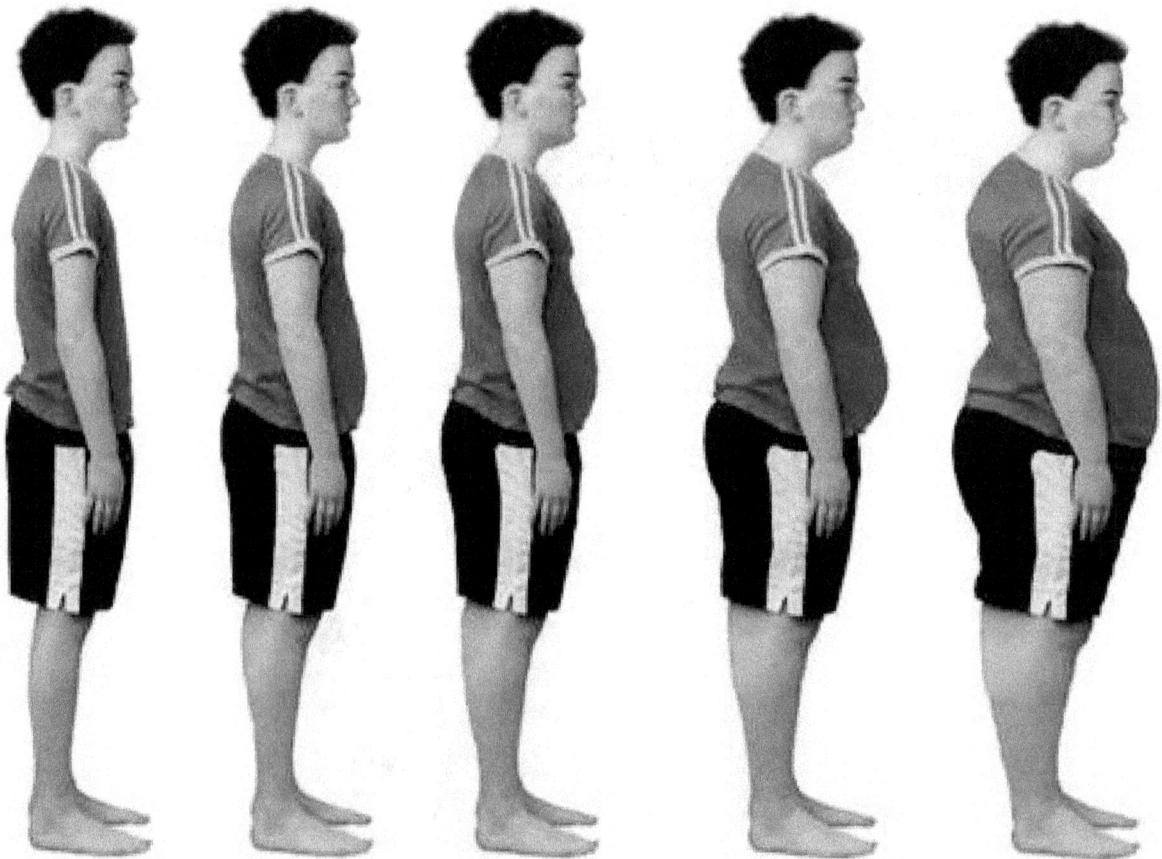

The levels of obesity are usually listed as marginally overweight, overweight, very overweight or obese, morbid obesity, and super obesity. Marginally overweight means you're just a few pounds more than you should be. Super obese means you probably weigh twice or more than you should. Since we are all different and the right weight for each of us is different, a more accurate way of telling whether you're unwholesomely fat is to measure your Body Mass Index. This is a little complicated to measure but your doctor could get your BMI number for you. A general scale to compare yourself to follows:

Women	Men
Marginally Overweight: 25.8-27.3	26.4-27.8
Overweight or Obese: 27.3-32.3	27.8-31.1
Very Overweight: >32.3	>31.1

Morbid Obesity for both Women and Men: 40-49.9
Super Obesity for both Women and Men: >50

Problems with breathing could come with any of these levels of obesity but is less likely to come in the lower levels and much more likely to show up in the higher levels.

What you've suspected is asthma might be a simple need to lose a few pounds. Share your concerns with your doctor and together work out what is the real underlying problem.

Medicines Used to Treat Asthma

Asthma is a rather complicated disease involving the dysfunction of numerous cell types. The resulting condition in an asthmatic lung requires several types of medicines for effective treatment. Let's discuss the two primary classes of medicines used and the different types of medicines in each class.

Long Term Control Medicines

The first of the two primary classes of medicines used in the treatment of asthma is the long term control medicines. Let's quickly revisit the Expert Panel's definition of asthma:

*Asthma is a chronic **inflammatory disorder of the airways** in which many cells and cellular elements play a role: in particular, mast cells, eosinophils, neutrophils (especially in sudden onset, fatal exacerbations, occupational asthma, and patients who smoke), T lymphocytes, macrophages, and epithelial cells. In susceptible individuals, this inflammation causes recurrent episodes of coughing (particularly at night or early in the morning), wheezing, breathlessness, and chest tightness. These episodes are usually associated with widespread but variable airflow obstruction that is often reversible either spontaneously or with treatment.*

Notice the words in bold letters--inflammatory disorder of the airways. The objective of medicines classified as long term control medicines is to provide better control of asthma by reducing the inflammation and swelling in the airways. The medicines who make this list are effective to some degree at doing this. The medicine found to be most effective at managing inflammation is corticosteroids.

Corticosteroids

Corticosteroids are anti-inflammatory medicines which have been found to reduce the over-excitability of the airways. This tendency of the airway to get over excited, referred to as hyper-responsive, is the beginning point of flareups. Corticosteroids tend to dampen this hyper-responsive nature of the airway.

During an asthma attack, certain cells rush to the site of the airway disturbance (something like what police do). Corticosteroids slow this influx of these inflammatory cells and thereby lessen the degree of inflammation that occurs.

Corticosteroids can be given as injections, as liquids or pills, or can even be inhaled. Corticosteroids are the most effective of all the medicines included in the long term control medicine category and is sold under many names. A short list includes Budesonide (sold as Pulmicort), Triamcinolone acetonide (sold as Azmacort and discontinued as of 12/31/2009), and Mometasone (sold as Asmanex). Inhaled corticosteroids (ICSs) are often prescribed for longterm control as they are known to reduce the likelihood of flare-ups and when flare-ups do occur to limit how bad those flare-ups get. A few names of inhaled steroids include Fluticasone, Flunisolide, Mometasone, and Beclomethasone. Below are some images of inhaled steroids used for long term control of asthma.

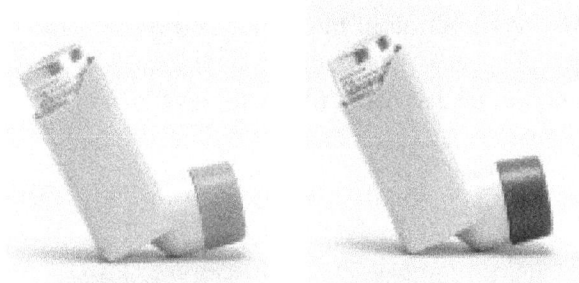

images curtesy of Michael J. Schumacher

The above two images are curtesy of Michael J. Schumacher, MB, FRACP of the University of Arizona, are of mint flavored Flunisolide (Aerobid-M) and regular Flunisolide (Aerobid). Complaints of bad taste encouraged the development of the mint flavored version. Aerobid has fallen out of favor somewhat since patients won't take it as often as they should due to bad taste.

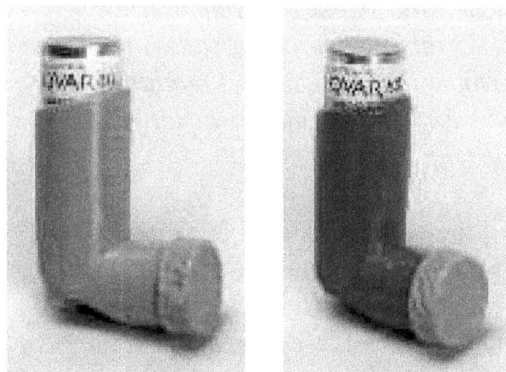

images curtesy of Michael J. Schumacher

Both of the above images are Beclomethasone. The brownish colored canister is Beclomethasone (Qvar 40). The maroon colored inhaler is Qvar 80. The numbers 40 and 80 refer to the amount of medicine in each puff.

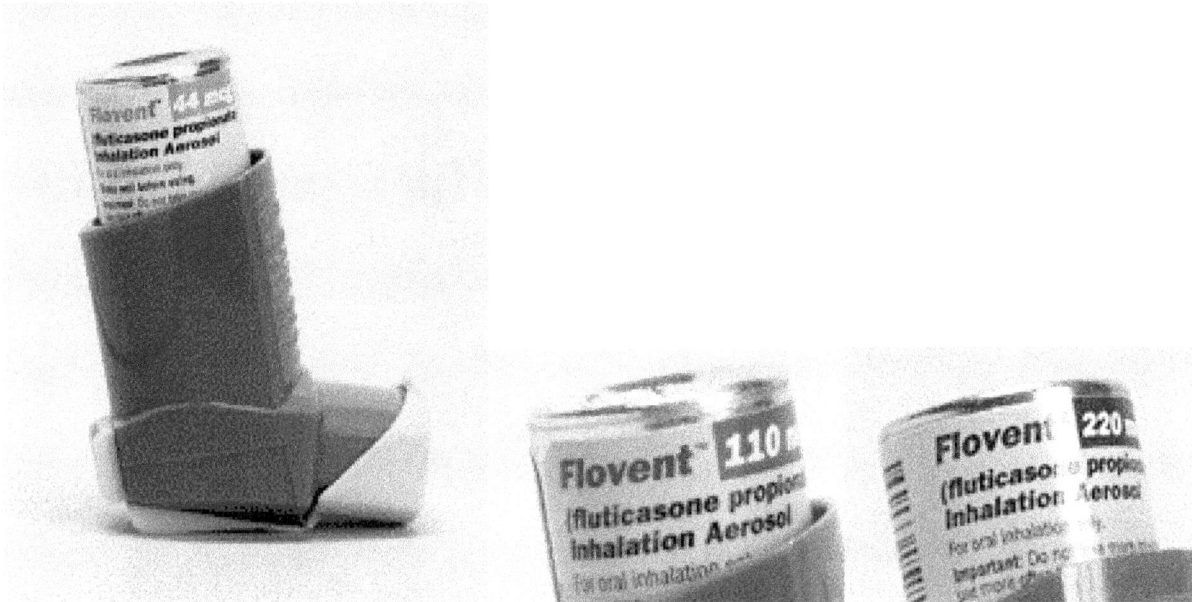

images curtesy of Michael J. Schumacher

These are images of fluticasone propionate. Fluticasone comes in several strengths and can also be found in diskus form. These are in MDI (metered dose inhaler) form under the name of Flovent.

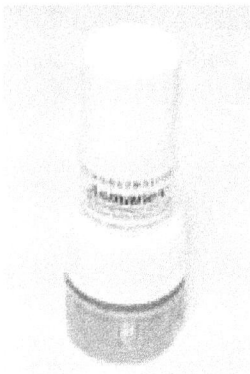

images curtesy of Michael J. Schumacher

This image of mometasone (sold as Asmanex) is in the form of what is called a twisthaler. These steroids shown here are only a few of the many available. You and your doctor can decide which of these or other steroids will work best for you.

A new corticosteroid which has relatively recently come to market is ciclesonide and is sold under the name of Alvesco.

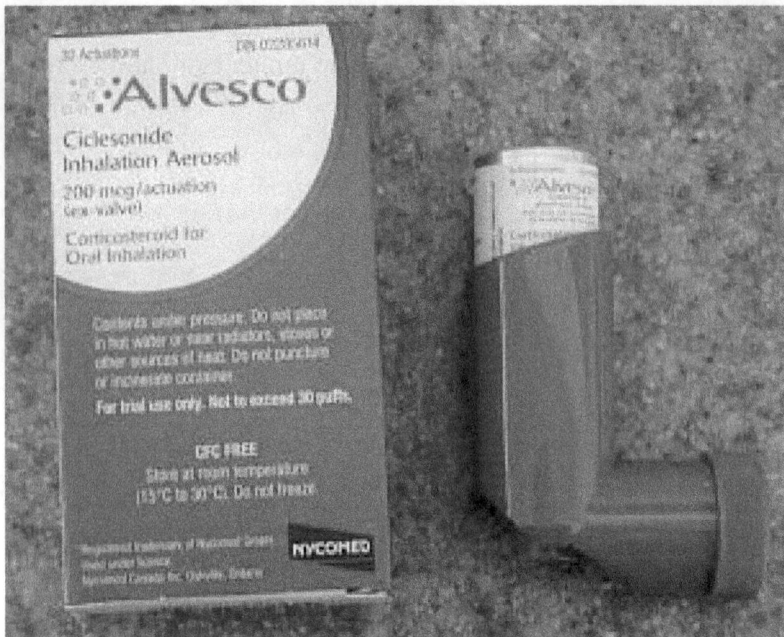

This steroid is said to be less likely to cause oral thrush. If other steroids have been a problem for you, ask your doctor or pharmacist about ciclesonide.

  It would be smart practice to rinse your mouth after using it just as you would with other inhaled steroids.

IMPORTANT: You should take all medicines just as your doctor directs. Here are a few things to remember about steroids:

Steroids are control medicines and are meant to help *prevent* asthma attacks. Once an attack has started, steroids will not stop the attack. Inhaled steroids could even make an attack worse if given during the attack. It will take another type of medicine (quick-relief medicine) to stop the attack. Your doctor will try to find the lowest dose possible to effectively help with your asthma. His goal is to control your asthma without causing unwanted side effects. Among the side effects are cough, hoarse voice, or oral thrush (fungal infection in the mouth).

Remember to always rinse your mouth after taking an inhaled steroid. If you rinse or brush your teeth after taking an inhaled steroid, you'll be less likely to have side effects from the medicine.

Cromolyn Sodium and Nedocromil

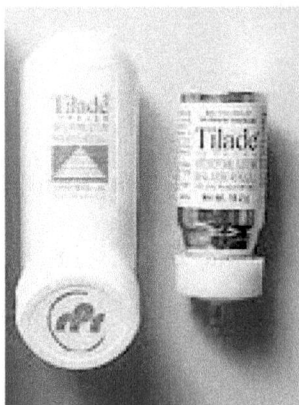

An image of Nedocromil Sodium sold under the name of Tilade.

Here is the definition of asthma again.

*Asthma is a chronic inflammatory disorder of the airways in which many cells and cellular elements play a role: in particular, **mast cells**, eosinophils, neutrophils (especially in sudden onset, fatal exacerbations, occupational asthma, and patients who smoke), T lymphocytes, macrophages, and epithelial cells. In susceptible individuals, this inflammation causes recurrent episodes of coughing (particularly at night or early in the morning), wheezing, breathlessness, and chest tightness. These episodes are usually associated with widespread but variable airflow obstruction that is often reversible either spontaneously or with treatment.*

There are several things that happen during an asthma attack. Think of those several things as links in a chain. If you can break any of those links in the chain involved in causing the attack then you can limit how bad the attack is or prevent it altogether.

These two medicines help to limit inflammation in the airways by stabilizing certain cells involved in inflammation.

During the series of steps leading to swelling and inflammation, some cells burst open and release substances which play a big role in the swelling of the airway. Cromolyn Sodium (once sold under the name Intal but no longer available) stabilizes those cells (called mast cells) and prevents them from bursting open. Nedocromil (sold as Tilade and no longer available since 6/14/10) helps the airway in that same way--by helping to prevent the mast cells from bursting open and releasing those substances which leads to swelling and inflammation of the airway.

Immunomodulators

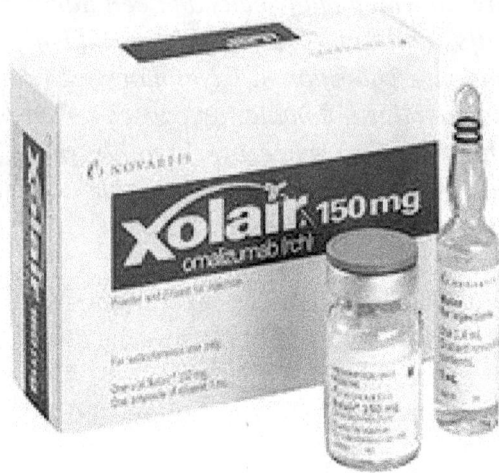

These medicines are fairly new in the fight against asthma. The name of these medicines say it all: immuno- relates to the immune system and -modulate means to change the strength of something. In the case of asthma, this medicine wants to change the strength of the immune response by weakening it. Remember how the asthmatic airway overreacts to stimulants? This overreaction is the immune system's overreaction. Immunomodulators try to get the immune system to calm down. It encourages the immune system to take a chill pill.

Omalizumab helps those asthmatics who have allergies that make their asthma worse. For example, allergies to dust mites, mold, or animal dander.

Omalizumab (Xolair is the name it's sold under and it's pronounced as Zo-Lair) is the medicine in this group of medicines found to be most helpful in fighting allergic asthma. Xolair is given as an injection but only to severe asthmatics who are twelve years of age and older. It doesn't happen often but this medicine can cause severe allergic reactions called anaphylactic shock which could be life threatening. So, if your doctor considers you a good candidate to be helped by Xolair, this is a risk that you and your doctor should be very aware of.

Leukotriene modifiers

So that you don't have to flip back to look at the definition of asthma, here it is again.

*Asthma is a chronic inflammatory disorder of the airways in which many cells and cellular elements play a role: in particular, **mast cells**, **eosinophils**, neutrophils (especially in sudden onset, fatal exacerbations, occupational asthma, and patients who smoke), T lymphocytes, macrophages, and epithelial cells. In susceptible individuals, this inflammation causes recurrent episodes of coughing (particularly at night or early in the morning), wheezing, breathlessness, and chest tightness. These episodes are usually associated with widespread but variable airflow obstruction that is often reversible either spontaneously or with treatment.*

The bold words are those cell types interfered with by this type of long term control medicine. Without the interference, the asthma attack would develop in it's usual way. With the interference, the pathway of events which leads to the attack is blocked somewhat.

There are two primary medicines in this group; Leukotriene receptor antagonists (referred to as LTRAs) and 5-lipoxygenase inhibitors.

Montelukast (sold under the name of Singulair) is the most used medicine of the LTRAs. It's an easy pill to swallow since the usual prescription is just one pill a day. The image below shows this pill front and back at several times it's normal size.

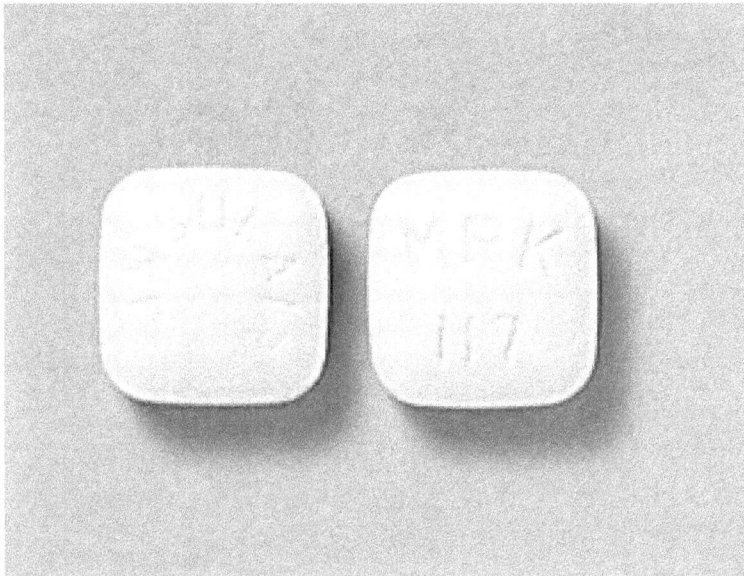
Singulair pillsS

The 5-lipoxygenase inhibitor is sold under the name of Zyflo. Zyflo is not as popular since you have to be twelve years old or older to take the pill and it has to be taken four times a day. It also can affect your liver so your doctor has to keep his eye on that too.

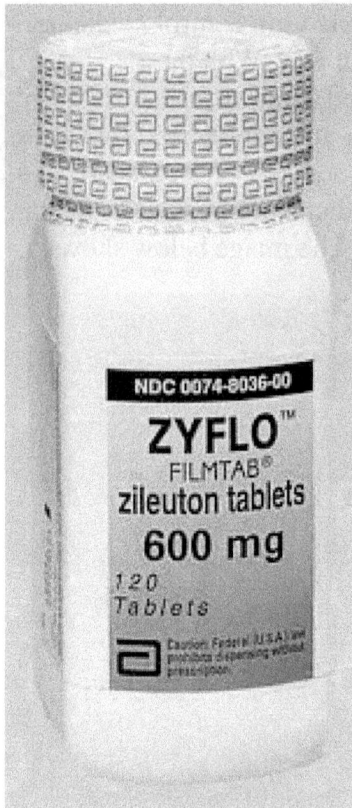

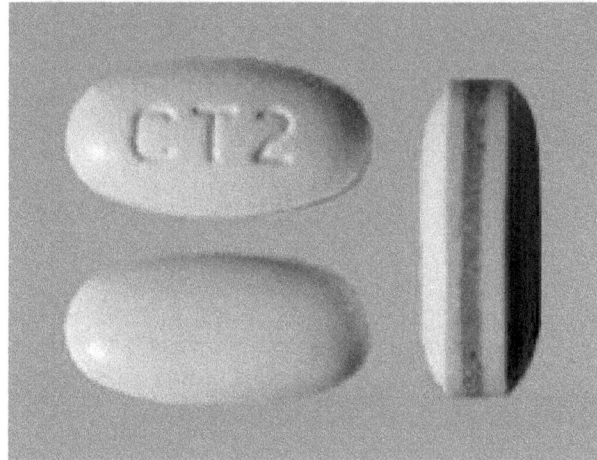

Zyflo pills

Long Acting Beta Agonists (LABA)

LABAs are long acting bronchodilators. Short acting beta agonists like Albuterol or Levalbuterol are the medicines to use when you're having an attack. LABAs are not used in that way. LABAs are used to help *prevent* attacks. A couple of examples of this medicine is Salmeterol (sold as Serevent) and Formoterol (sold as Foradil).

Salmeterol in Diskus and MDI forms

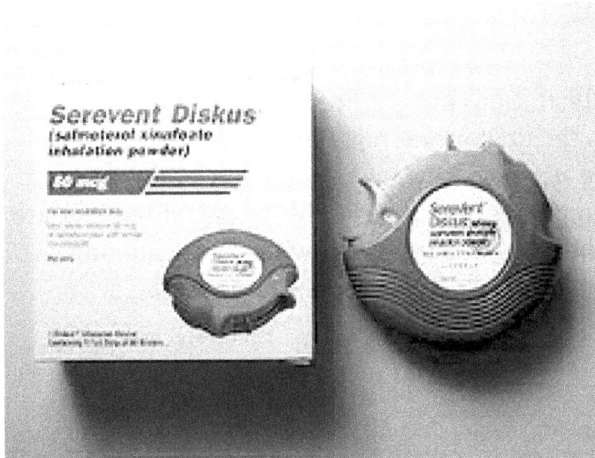

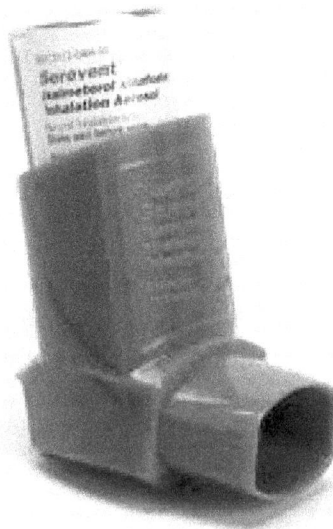

Salmeterol is sold under the name Serevent

Formoterol is sold under the name Foradil. The image below is the Foradil Aerolizer.

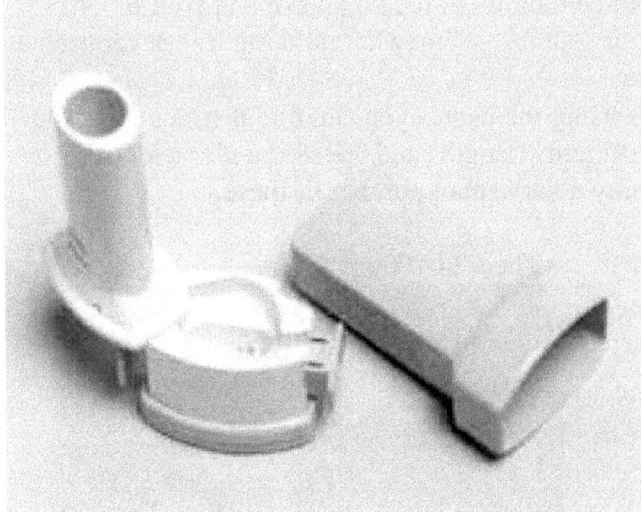

The image below is Foradil as a Turbuhaler.

IMPORTANT: Directions on how to use these devices will be given later in this book.

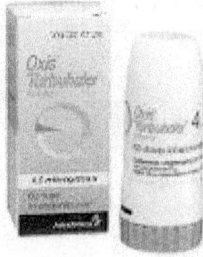

IMPORTANT: The FDA (Food and Drug Administration) has warned you to be careful when taking this medicine. It is perfectly safe if taken as the doctor orders it but it could cause your death if you do not. Long Acting Beta Agonists are **never** to be used as your only control medicine. It should always be used **with** another control medicine, usually steroids. Frequent use of a LABA during times of troubled breathing could make it hard to tell when your asthma is getting worse. Remember to get frequent checkups if your doctor has prescribed a long acting beta agonist for you.

Methylxanthines

There are a number of medicines in this group of long-term control medicines but only Theophylline is included in the Expert Panel's third report on asthma. Theophylline is a mild to moderate bronchodilator used as an alternative long term control medicine for its anti-inflammatory effects. It is a medicine that has to be monitored for toxic levels in your blood. Theophylline can be useful as a treatment if your asthma is somewhat mild but it is never used as a control medicine when asthma is more severe.

Below are some images of Theophylline pills using the names you can find them under at the drug store. Theophylline pills come in many different strengths and are sold under a lot of different names. The images below represent only a very small number of these.

Quibron 300 mg

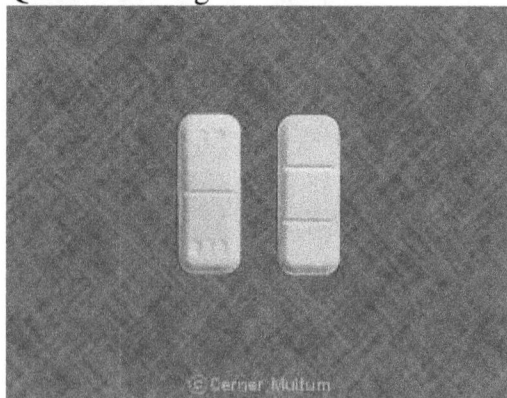

Theo-24 100 mg

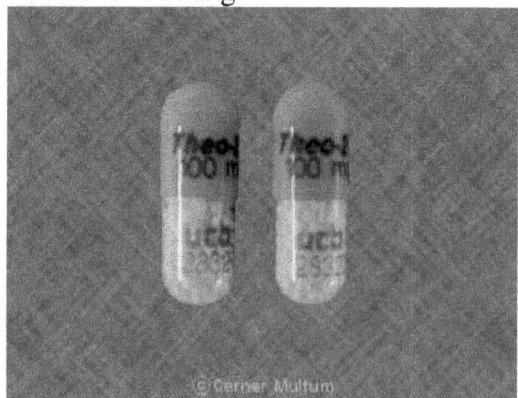

Theo-Dur 200 mg

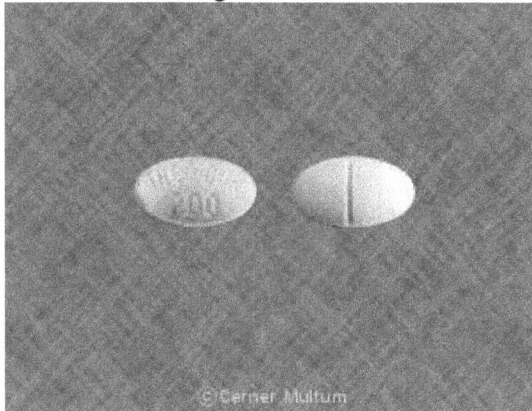

Combination Inhalers

Some drug manufacturers have combined two different medicines into one inhaler. These combination inhalers often have steroids and long acting beta agonists as the active medicines.

The benefits of these inhalers are that two of the primary issues of asthma can be treated at the same time. The long acting beta agonist will treat smooth muscle constriction while the steroid treats inflammation.

Symbicort and Advair are two popular such medicines. Symbicort contains the steroid budesonide and the LABA formoterol. Advair contains the steroid fluticasone and the LABA (long acting beta agonist) salmeterol.

A new medicine which has come to market at about the time of this writing is called Dulera. Dulera contains the steroid mometasone and the LABA formoterol.

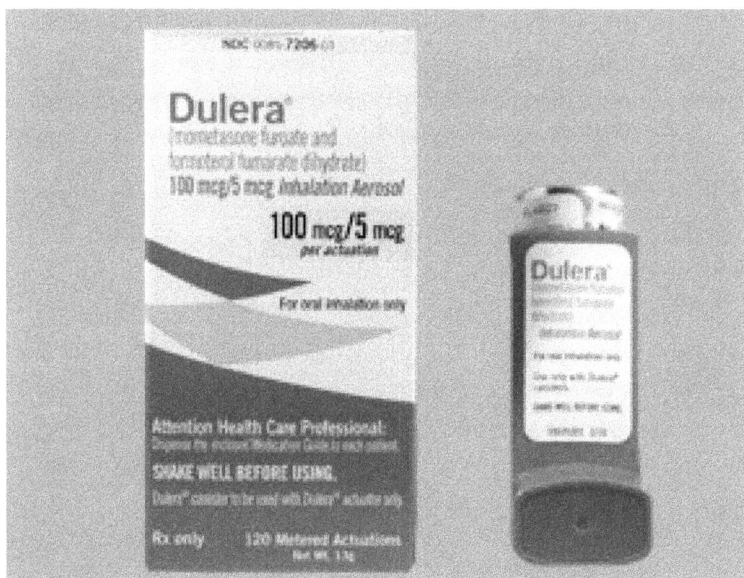

Both the steroid and the LABA of each of these combination inhalers are sold as single medicine inhalers also. Of the steroids, budesonide is sold as Pulmicort, mometasone is sold as Asmanex and fluticasone is sold as Flovent. Of the long acting beta agonists, salmeterol is sold as Serevent and formoterol is sold as Foradil.

You should treat these medicines as you would your other inhalers. Take them as prescribed. Side effects would be hoarseness, throat irritation, tremors or increased heart rate. A combination of the effects you can expect from steroids and beta agonists. Since these combination inhalers contain steroids, remember to rinse your mouth after each use.

Check with your doctor about a prescription for a combination medicine if you think it would work well for you.

Quick-Relief Medicines

The second of the two primary classes of medicines used to treat asthma is the quick-relief medicines. This group is called 'quick-relief' because they are used during an attack to give you some quick relief from your distress. There are a number of medicines in this class but let's talk about the one in this group that is most widely used.

Short Acting Beta Agonists

The most popular of these short acting beta agonists are albuterol, levalbuterol, and pirbuterol. These short acting beta agonists(called SABAs for short) open the airway and improve breathing during times of chest tightness and trouble breathing by relaxing the muscle that surrounds the airway. They are called beta agonists because they activate certain sites in the lung called 'beta receptors.' Beta receptors in the lungs, when activated, cause the muscle surrounding the airway to relax. When the muscle relaxes, the air passageway gets bigger and you can breath more easily.

Albuterol is made available by numerous drug companies and is called by lots of different names; Pro-Air, Ventolin, Proventil and many others. Levalbuterol is sold under the name of Xopenex and can be found as an MDI or as a liquid for nebulization. Pirbuterol can be found under the name of Maxair. Below are some images of several of these medicines. These images are **curtesy of Michael J. Schumacher** of the University of Arizona.

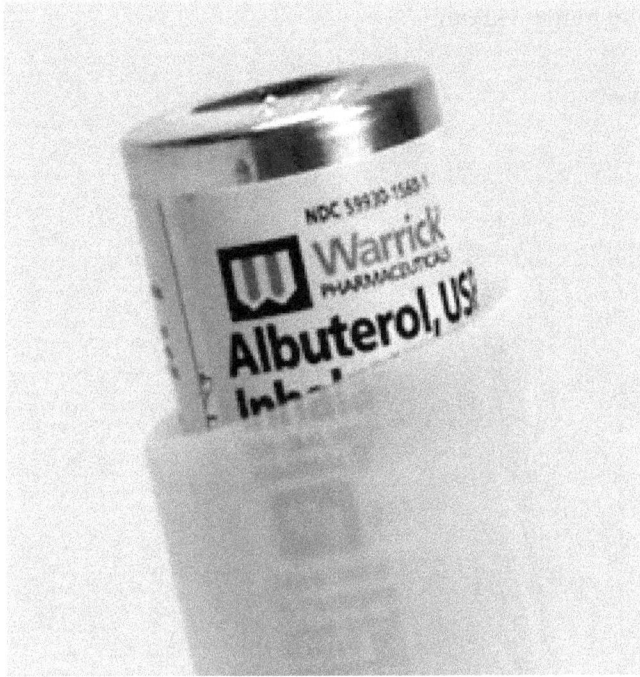

An image of generic albuterol MDI

An image of a Pro-Air MDI

An image of a Proventil MDI

A Ventolin MDI

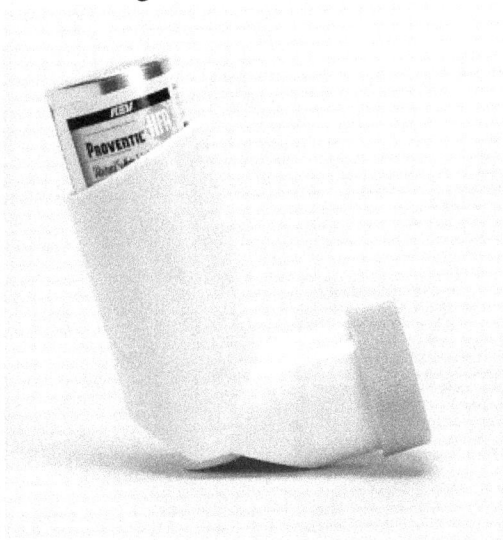

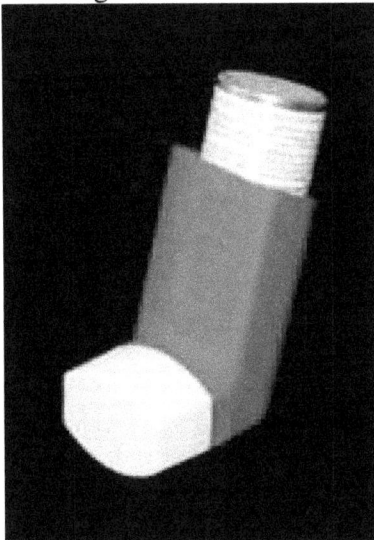

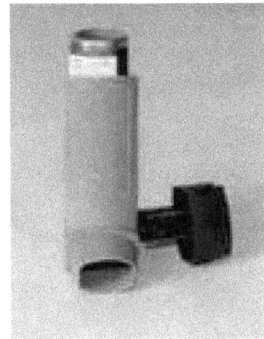

Images of pirbuterol. Pirbuterol is sold under the name Maxair.

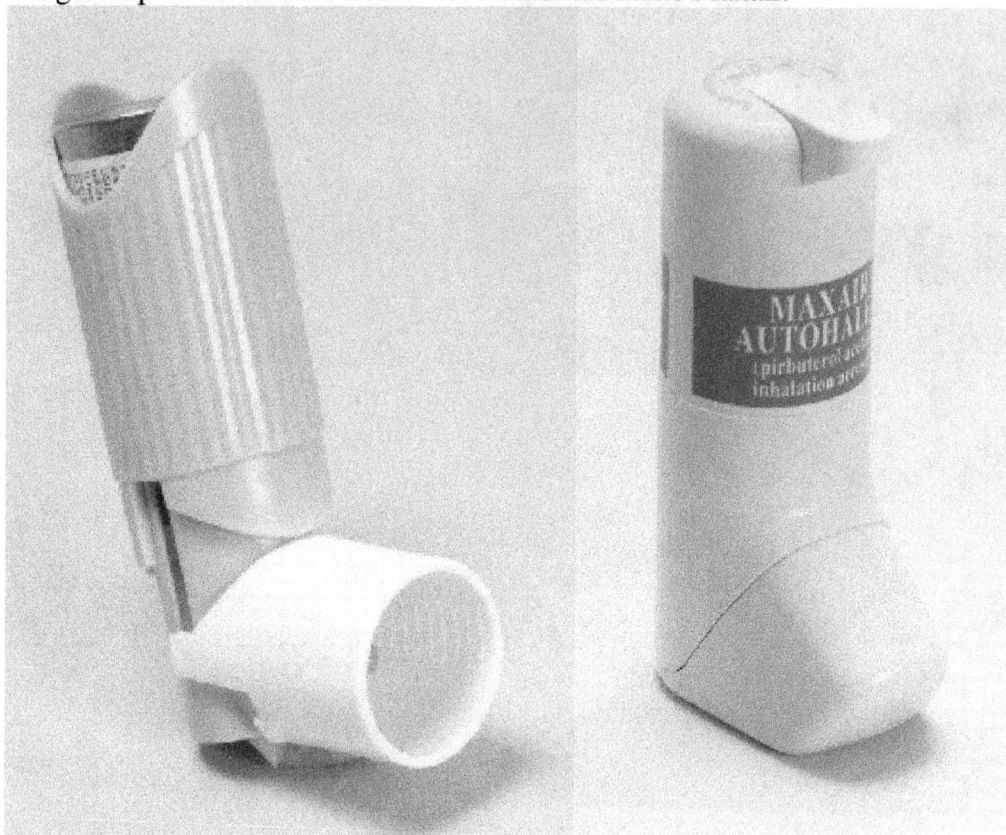

An image of levalbuterol under the name of Xopenex

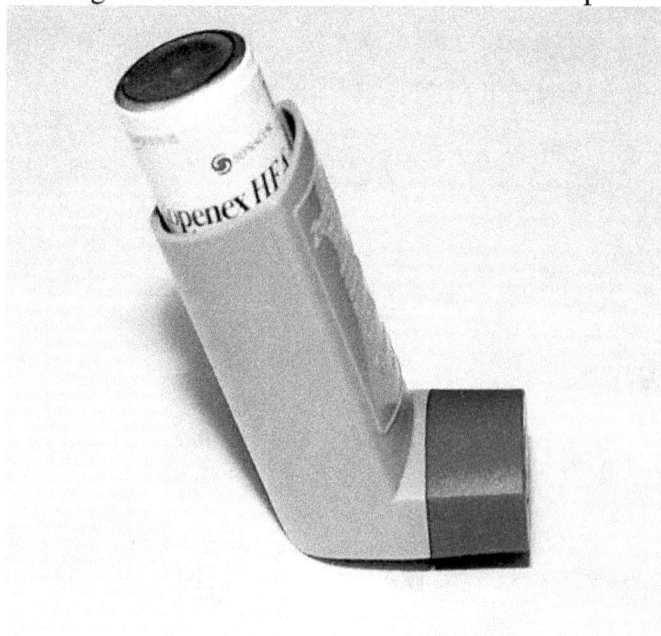

IMPORTANT: These medicines are very effective at giving quick relief from asthma attacks. It is important that you follow your doctors directions when taking these medicines. You can expect your heart to beat faster and you might become jittery. Albuterol is more likely to cause these 'side effects' than levalbuterol. When using an MDI always use an aerochamber. Aerochambers will limit your side effects by helping most of the medicine get to your lungs. Aerochambers and spacers will be discussed later in the book.

Anticholinergics

Anticholinergics also help open the airway for easier breathing. Where SABAs open the airway by activating beta receptors, anticholinergics open airways by blocking muscarinic receptors. The short story is it helps make it easier to breath during an attack. These medicines don't act as fast as SABAs but are still considered to be quick-relief medicines.

There are few side effects to worry about. Ipratropium bromide can potentially cause headache, tachycardia or nausea but these effects are rare. It can also dry your mouth and your secretions.

Generally anticholinergics are deemed more effective when combined with SABAs but they can be used alone. This medicine is also preferred if a sudden asthma attack is started by your use of some type of beta blocker (we'll discuss medicines that might cause attacks later).

Ipratropium Bromide is the most common anticholinergic used for asthma and the only one mentioned in the Expert Panel's report. Ipratropium is sold under the names Atrovent, Apovent, and Aerovent. Ipratropium can be found in MDI or liquid form. Below are images of ipratropium bromide in MDI and liquid forms under the name of Atrovent.

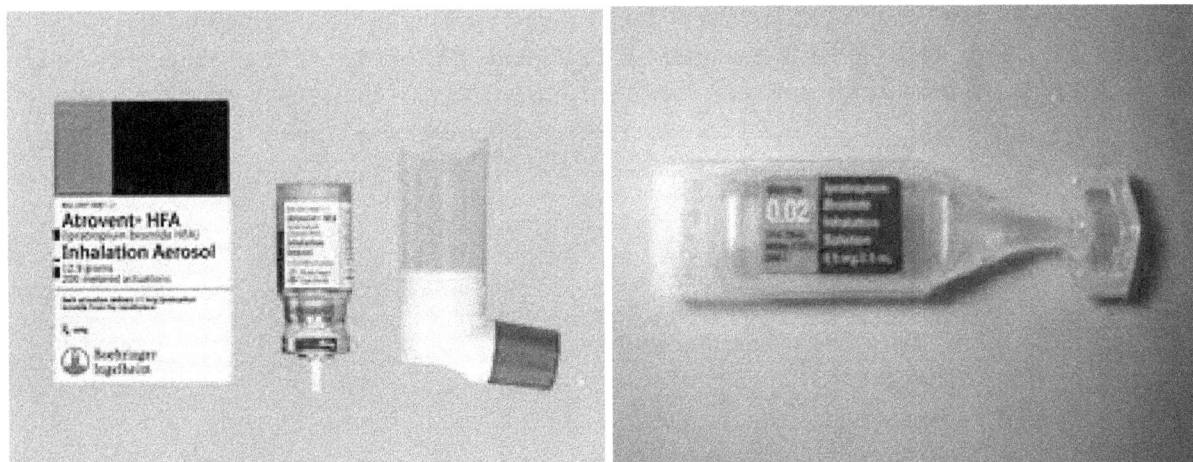

Systemic Corticosteroids

Now, it might seem confusing that corticosteroids are considered a long term control medicine and a quick-relief medicine but this is how you can keep that straight. A long term control corticosteroid is usually the inhaled corticosteroids like Flovent, Aerobid, or Qvar. These medicines are used to help prevent attacks and to help control how bad those attacks get. These *inhaled* steroids are used everyday, sometimes for months, depending on how well your asthma is being controlled. They are not used to help you reverse an attack.

Systemic steroids *are* used to help you reverse an attack. They are often given as a shot or they can be swallowed as pills or liquid. The systemic corticosteroids help you return to normal faster. The inflammation that is part of the reason for the attack is reduced by systemic steroids.

Systemic steroids are prescribed infrequently and over short periods. Periods of seven to ten days are common. A short list of some systemic steroids are Prednisone, Prednisolone and Methylprednisolone. Since systemic steroids can come in a hundred different pill shapes and colors, here is just one image of the steroid Prednisone:

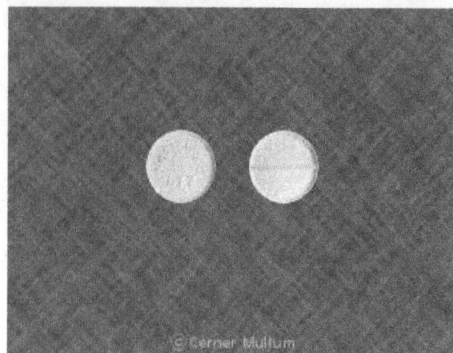

Prednisone and the other systemic steroids comes in different strengths. Always follow your doctor's directions when systemic steroid pills or liquids are prescribed.

Trigger Avoidance and Control

Triggers are those things that cause your asthma to flare up. Triggers can be practically anything. If it can be identified as the cause of your attacks, it is a trigger. Triggers can be found indoors or outdoors, at work or at home. Triggers can even be an emotion like extreme anger. Let's discuss some triggers so you can become more aware of what could be behind some of your attacks.

Indoor Triggers

Now that we know what a trigger is, let's consider a few triggers that could be found inside your house and how you could learn to avoid them.

Smoke

Smoking is a universal trigger. Almost every asthmatic can have an attack triggered by smoke. If you intentionally inhale cigarette, pipe or cigar smoke directly into your lungs, you will almost certainly trigger an attack. Smoking can be an easily avoided trigger in some cases. If you're voluntarily smoking, quit. Your problem with that trigger is over.

Of course sometimes you don't have that much control over your exposure to the smoke. If the smoker in your home isn't you, you'll have less control over your exposure to smoke. Ask the smoker to please smoke outside and that will limit your exposure to smoke. Smoking in another

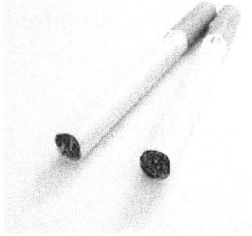

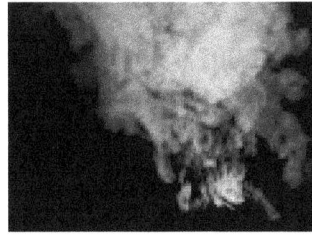

room in the house never works. The smoke will waft through all the rooms eventually so you'll be eventually exposed. To see how smoking anywhere inside will eventually cover everywhere inside, consider this: A pitcher of clear cool water. A dropper of ink. Select any point in the pitcher and drop one drop of ink. Eventually there will be no place within the pitcher where there is clear water untainted by ink. It is the same way with smoke in a house.

Smoking outside is the next best think to quitting when trying to limit an asthmatic's exposure to smoke. There is even a 'most effective' way to smoke outside to avoid carrying smoke back inside on clothing and in hair. When you smoke outside, wear a head covering and a 'smoking shirt or jacket' that you leave outside. You should never wear the smoking garment back inside after smoking since you'll limit the effectiveness of this smoke avoidance step.

Dust Mites

Dust mites are sometimes the cause of asthma attacks. An allergist can help you determine if you're allergic to them. Dust mites are microscopic (you need a microscope to see them). These creatures infest most peoples' beds, pillows, sheets and other bed clothes. They feed on skin flakes we all lose in bed. If you're allergic to them, you'll find that your asthma will give you more trouble after your exposure to them. You'll wheeze more and will likely wake up at night with chest tightness and trouble breathing more often. Dust mites are virtually unavoidable but exposure to them can be limited.

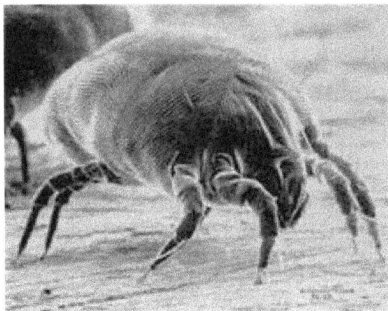

If it is determined that you are allergic to dust mites, you can limit your exposure to them by doing just a few little things.

Look for a dust mite cover for your pillows, box spring and mattress. These covers will prevent you from breathing in the mites and their fecal matter which is really the allergen that causes all the trouble for you. The pore size of the covers is between three and five microns, too small for even a dust mite to get through. Think of how long an inch is then slice that inch into about 400,000 pieces and one of those pieces is approximately the length of a micron. Google dust mite covers and explore this way of limiting your exposure.

Wash your bedding weekly in hot water. Temperatures between 130 and 150 degrees Fahrenheit will kill dust mites. If it's bedding you can't wash, freeze it. Putting bedding in the freezer overnight will kill dust mites too.

Consider trading in your window drapes for blinds. Dust mites are less at home on plastic blinds than on heavy cloth drapes. Try to keep the dust cleaned off your furniture but do it with a damp cloth so the dust won't get up into the air.

Dust mites need water to survive. If you deny them their moisture, you'll limit their numbers. Dehumidify your sleeping space with an air conditioner or dehumidifier and you'll put a serious cramp in a dust mite's life. Your goal is a humidity level of 50% or less.

These techniques will help reduce the effect of dust mites on your asthma.

Animal Dander

Animal dander can be a major cause of asthma attacks.

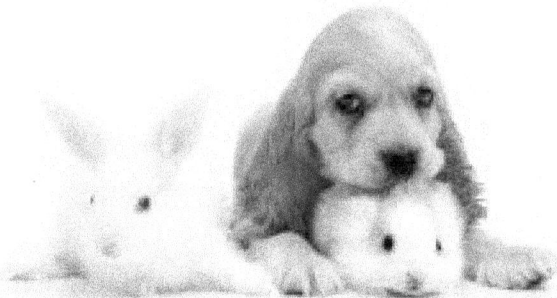

If you have a dog, cat or even a feathered pet, there is dander in your home. Contrary to what is sometimes believed, it isn't just the hair of a pet that causes the problem. Dander is from the proteins in your pet's saliva, urine, skin flakes, and feces. These proteins float through your home settling on your furniture, your bedding, and you. When the dander enters your respiratory system (unavoidable since you're breathing all the time there) you suffer increased breathing problems if you're allergic.

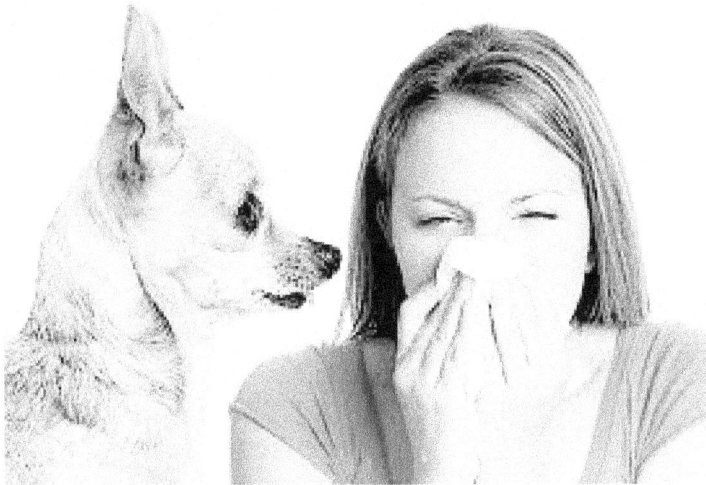

The ideal solution is to get rid of the pet. Since the dander is widespread throughout your home, it will take several months for dander levels to fall noticeably. If parting with the pet is too traumatic for you, following a few 'dander control' steps will be the next best thing.

Give your pet a bath regularly. This one step can do much to limit dry, flaking skin debris. Remember to allow the nonallergic member to do the bathing.

Keep your pet out of the bed room and off the bedding. On average you'll spend at least a third of your 24 hour days in your bed. Your asthma will be better controlled if those hours are mostly dander free.

If you will limit the area your pet is allowed to roam, you'll reduce the area where extra cleaning would be needed to control the dander.

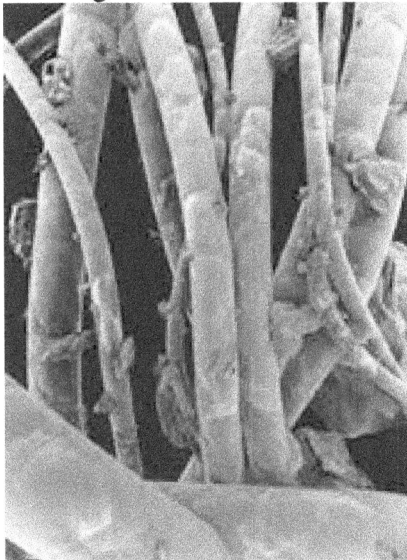

An image of animal hairs and skin (dyed for easier viewing)

Hard surfaced floors like hardwood or linoleum would be easier to keep more dander free than a carpet would be. If you have carpet and you're able to switch to a hard surface flooring, your asthma will thank you for it. If you must deal with the carpeted floors you have, using a filter in your vacuum cleaner will limit your dander exposure (allow the nonallergic member to vacuum).

HEPA air purifiers are also helpful in reducing the amount of dander allergens in a home. Some claim to be over 99% effective in filtering dander from the air.

If all these precautions and suggestions are put into practice, you'll be well on your way to better controlling your asthma.

Molds

It's hard to get away from some things that is bad for your asthma. Molds are one of those things. Most people can breathe molds in and out all day without any ill effects but asthmatics with mold allergies cannot. Mold can cause wheezing, irritated eyes, stuffy nose and sometimes rashes if you have a mold allergy. Types of molds that are usually to blame for aggravating allergic asthmatics are Alternaria, *Cladosporium, Penicillium, and Aspergillus.*

mold under a sink

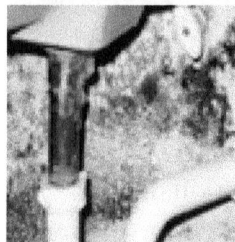

mold on grout

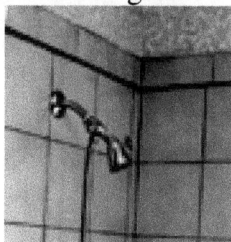

mold on shower curtain

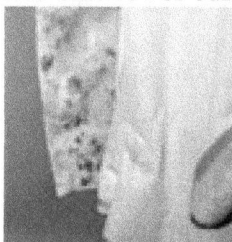

mold on sliding door seal

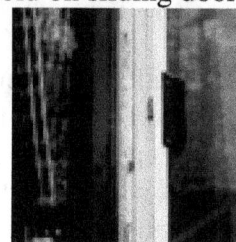

Molds are fungi and they're spread by tiny seeds called spores. Spores float around on air in your house until they land on something damp where they can grow. They grow best in dark, dank, warm places like basements, old garbage cans, and shower stalls.

Warm moist places make molds right at home. If you want to make it difficult for mold to grow, you have to control the moisture.

Make sure you leave no standing water. Dry the shower stall well after use. If a water leak is discovered, get it repaired right away. Remember that warmth and moisture is great if you're trying to grow mold. If you're trying to discourage the growth of mold, control the moisture in your house.

Roaches

Believe it or not, roaches can cause allergic reactions in some people. If you get a stuffy nose that just won't go away or if your 'asthma season' seems to never end, you probably have an allergy to something and it could be roaches.

Certain proteins in a roaches saliva and feces can be the cause of your allergy. Even their body parts like legs or torsos could be the cause of your allergic reactions.

American Cockroach

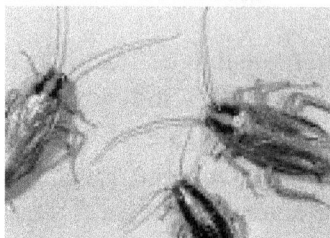

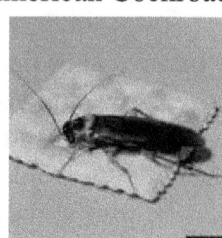

American Cockroach

Roaches are very tough survivalists so don't feel bad if you have some. They are really hard to get rid of but since their likes and dislikes are known, it can be done.

You have to get rid of their food, their water, and their hiding places. If you keep your stovetop and counter tops clean, that will help in getting rid of their food. You should also be sure to keep the kitchen floor clean since food sometimes falls unnoticed to the floor. Make sure you wash your dishes after eating or you'll be feeding the Roach family too. Don't leave food out after a meal and cover it with tightly fitted lids or aluminum foil. They'll eat almost anything including paint chips and newspapers so you can't allow stacks of newspaper or junk mail to pile up.

Standing water in the sink, leaky faucets or sweating pipes will provide the water they need. If you can limit their water supply you can encourage them to find somewhere else to live. They like to hang out where it's warm and wet and where there's something to eat.

While you're making it hard for them to find water and food and a comfortable place to live, you can be killing them too. Try baits or traps to reduce their numbers. These methods are less hurtful to your asthma. If you must use a pesticide spray, try to get someone else to do the spraying.

Cockroaches are hard to evict but it can be done. You might find that your asthma improves after these steps are put into practice.

Indoor Plants

Indoor plants present less of an allergic threat than outdoor plants but you still have to be mindful of them. Christmas trees can be a problem for some asthmatics since they can carry mold. Actually, mold can develop in the bottom of the pot of any indoor plant.

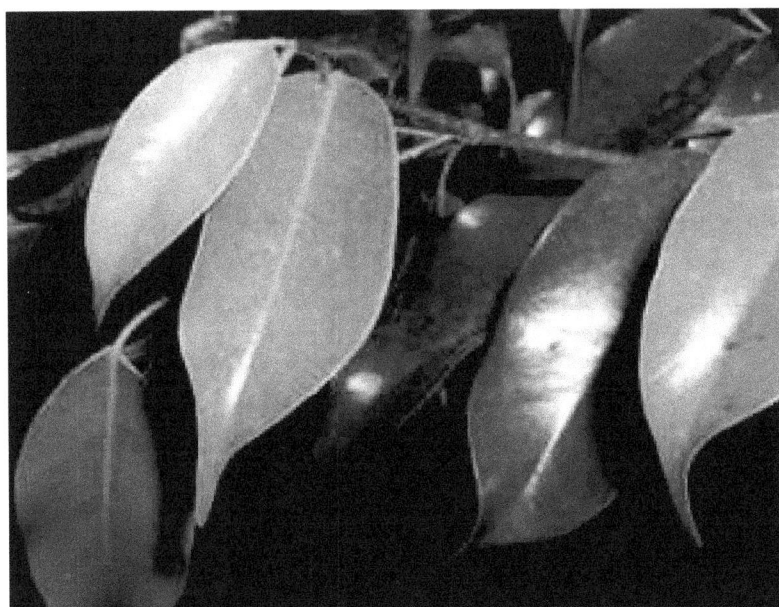
Weeping Fig

Certain plants like the weeping fig (which can irritate the eyes) or the flowering maple (which can directly affect the airways) are specifically allergenic.

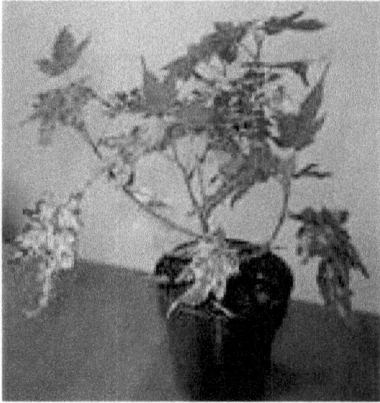

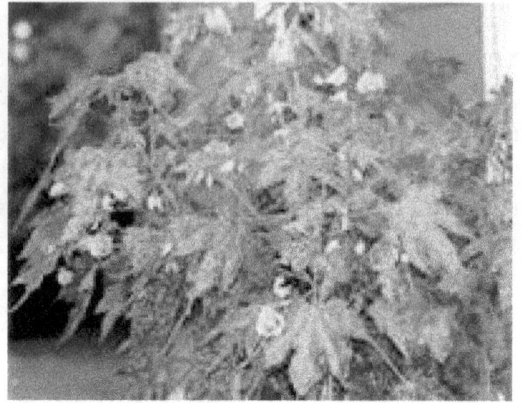

Flowering Maples

Any flowering plant will have to pollenate and could cause you problems with its pollen.

Plants sometimes collect dust and the dust could be a starting point for problems with dust mites.

So you even have to be careful with *plants* if you want to minimize your exposure to indoor allergens.

Outdoor Triggers

Just as there are indoor dangers to your asthma, there are also outdoor dangers. You'll find yourself a little less able to control the outdoor triggers but there are still things you can do to protect yourself. The most important thing is to become aware of the risk, then you can devise ways to limit it.

Planning when and when not to go outside is a big part of remaining symptom free. When you must be outside try to limit your exposure by watching where you go. You should also attempt to remove those triggers from your skin as soon and completely as possible.

Outside smoke can be a trigger to an attack just as surely as inside smoke. Avoid being near burning debris, leaves and the like. Smoke from grills can cause asthma attacks too. You can eat grilled food without doing the grilling as smoke from grills can certainly be trouble for your asthma.

Most of your problems from outdoor triggers will be from molds and pollens.

Image of mold spores

Image of pollen

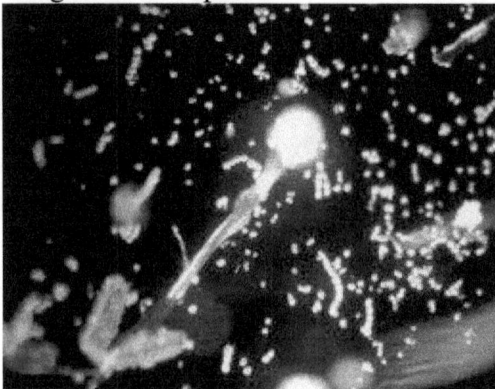

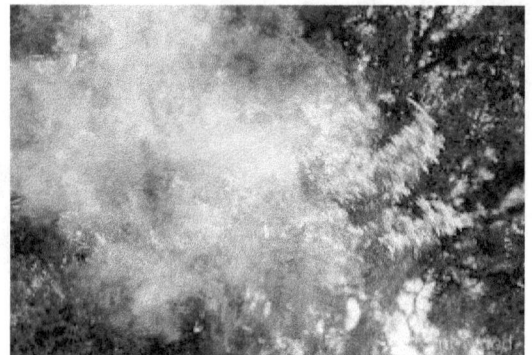

You can't see these microscopic seeds to avoid them. You'll just have to know your environment to know what type of triggers are out there and when they'll be out there.

Mold spores are usually heavy early in the year, around springtime. Pollen will usually peak between July and October.

It does matter when you go outside. On wet or cloudy days the pollen count is usually lower. The lower the pollen count the less likely you'll have a flare-up. When the wind is high and the weather is hot and dry, the air is full of pollen. This is a time when you should avoid going outside if possible.

Since plants are major potential triggers, avoid going near wooded areas where there are many plants. Gardens, especially flower gardens, should be avoided.

Your lawn might have to be cut if you have one but you should avoid being the one who cuts it. This could be a major cause of breathing problems. Ask a family member or pay someone to do your yard work or consider changing your green grass for a southwestern US styled lawn--cacti. If you simply must do it yourself, wear a mask to limit how much pollen you breathe in.

It is important to exercise but if it can be done inside when there is pollen flying around outside, you'll be better off.

Do you have a compost pile? It's the perfect mold breeding ground. When you stir the pile or add to it, wear a mask capable of blocking much of the mold and you'll be protecting yourself from a mold triggered attack.

Place mats at your entrances to your home so you can trap some of the triggers before you get inside. It would help if you could occasionally wash those mats.

When you're back inside you should immediately change clothes and shower. This will limit the amount of pollen or mold spores inside your home and help you to avoid spreading them throughout your house.

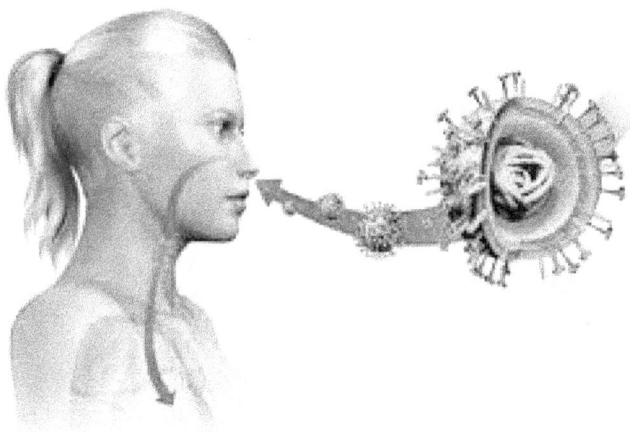

Rinse your nasal passages with warm saline water (Neti pots are great for this) to remove as many pollens as possible.

It is possible for you to escape the itchy, runny nose, excessive sneezing and congestion which usually come with exposure to these common outdoor allergens. You'll just have to be smart and plan when you go outside, where you go outside and what you do when you get back inside to win this outdoor trigger battle.

This list of indoor and outdoor triggers isn't complete. There are many more triggers both indoor and outdoor but it would be impossible to list them all. You've now been made aware of some common triggers and you can be careful to avoid other triggers when you've become aware of them. Just remember that whatever aggravates your asthma can be considered a trigger. Cold weather, strong emotions, exercise or anything else can be a trigger so be mindful of this and protect yourself from flare-ups as well as you can.

Asthma Action Plans and Assessment Tools

Asthma Action Plans

Asthma action plans have a simple goal: to help you manage your asthma. The plan does this by making sure that you understand how to take your daily medicines (if daily medicines have been prescribed), how to tell when your asthma is getting worse, what medicines to take when you notice you're getting worse, and how to tell when you should go to the doctor right away.

Let's consider the usual structure of an asthma action plan. The plan will usually have as its heading some information that you would like to find easily. Your doctor's phone number and name for example. Whatever other information you'd like to have quick and easy access to if your asthma starts getting bad, you'd like to have at the top of your action plan.

Next you would have your daily medicines listed. How much medicine you should take and how often you should take it. Usually these daily medicines are your control medicines. Your control medicines are typically your steroids.

Your quick-relief medicines would be listed next. How much medicine you should take and when you should take it. These medicines are the short acting beta agonists like albuterol. You take these medicines only if you're having some trouble. The plan would have the control medicines and quick-relief medicines separated for you to make it easy to understand.

Most action plans use the stoplight colors of green, yellow, and red to show you what to look for when your asthma is doing good (green), starting to do bad (yellow), and definitely doing bad (red). Each of the colors stands for how well you're doing. If you're in the green color or green zone, you're doing fine and should continue using the medicines just as your doctor wrote for you to use them when he gave them to you. If you're in the yellow zone you're starting to do bad and should change your medicine schedule a little. The asthma action plan should say exactly what you should change when you start to fit into a different zone. When you fit into the red zone there will be things you should change there too. Each zone will be a little bit different and it all depends on how well your asthma is treating you.

Each zone should show you what asthma symptoms fit into that zone. The green zone will say that you're not having any breathing trouble. You're not wheezing or coughing any more than you normally do and you're able to do the things that you're usually able to do. When you're in the green zone, you should just keep doing what your doctor has said for you to do and you'll be fine. The yellow zone will say that your wheezing and coughing has gotten a little worse. Your breathing is just a little more troubled than it usually is and you can't easily physically do what you've become used to doing. When you're in the yellow zone your asthma is getting worse and you should try to improve it if you can. The plan will tell you some things you should do to make your asthma get better. The red zone will say that your wheezing and coughing is now really bad. You can't easily physically do anything. Your distress is obvious to you and you should go to the emergency department for help. You should be following the instructions in the red zone of your asthma action plan as you go to the emergency department. You shouldn't wait because the red zone is telling you that your asthma has become critical.

If you use a peak flow (we will cover peak flows in a later chapter), the plan will list in each zone what peak flow value fits with that zone. The values might be shown as percentages instead of regular whole numbers. The green zone peak flow (PF) is eighty percent or better of your best PF. The yellow zone peak flow is from fifty percent to eighty percent of your best and the red zone PF is below fifty percent of the best that you usually do. The addition of this peak flow information will help those who use the peak flow meter to understand what to do when their peak flow numbers change.

The form below looks like an average action plan.

My Asthma Action Plan

Providers Name_____   My Name_____

Providers Number_____   Date_____

===

Controller Medicines	How much to take	How often	Other instructions
_____	_____	____ Times daily	Gargle and rinse afterwards
_____	_____	____ Times daily	
_____	_____	____ Times daily	

Quick-Relief Medicines	How much to take	How often	Other instructions
_____	_____	____ Times daily	If needing more often, see
_____	_____	____ Times daily	your doctor
_____	_____	____ Times daily	

==

Green Zone

I Feel Fine!

No problems breathing, My chest is not tight, I can easily do everything I usually do.

I will continue taking my controller medicine everyday as prescribed
I will take my quick-relief medicine whenever I need it but not on a schedule

==

Yellow Zone

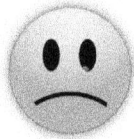

I Don't Feel So Good

I've started to have trouble breathing, My chest feels tight, I don't feel like my usual self

I will continue taking my controller medicine everyday as prescribed
I will take my quick-relief medicine now and in 20 minutes. If I feel better I'll take my quick-relief medicine every four hours for the next two days. If I don't feel better I'll take my quick-relief medicine again in 20 minutes then I'll call the doctor.

==

Red Zone

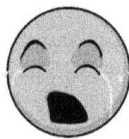

I Feel Horrible!

I can't seem to breath at all, My chest feels like an elephant is sitting on me, I need help

I'll take my quick-relief medicine at the high end of my dose range three times each 20 minutes
I'm going to the emergency department right now!

==
==

This is a typical asthma action plan. There can be many differences between plans but they should all have one thing in common: They should help you understand the difference between your control and quick-relief medicines, they should separate the zones by symptoms or peak flow readings, and they should help you recognize when your asthma is not good and tell you what you should do.

Everyone who has frequent trouble with their asthma or asthma that sometimes gets out of control should have an asthma action plan. To see how some other asthma action plans look, visit http://www.rampasthma.org/info-resources/asthma-action-plans/. You can also visit some of the resources in the last chapter of this book to view other action plans. Ask your doctor to help you get an asthma action plan if you often have trouble with your asthma or if it sometimes gets out of control.

Assessment Tools

Assessment tools are different from asthma action plans. Asthma action plans are guides to help you manage your asthma better. Assessment tools are tests to see if your asthma is being well managed.

Assessment tools can be designed for adults, kids, or a combination of adults and kids. These tests or series of questions try to answer the question 'Is my asthma under control?' There are usually just a few questions about things you would find easy to remember and to answer.

TRACK: Test for Respiratory and Asthma Control in Kids

TRACK is a test for preschool-aged children. It is for the doctor or other health care provider to complete. The TRACK test asks how often does your child have wheezing or coughing or trouble breathing, does your child seem able to play without getting out of breath, and how many times over the past month has your child awakened at night with trouble breathing. The first three question deals with symptoms and the final two questions deals with medicines. The TRACK test asks about how much quick-relief medicine you've used within the last three months and about oral steroid use over the past year.

You can see an example of this TRACK test in an article of the magazine Pediatrics at http://pediatrics.aappublications.org/content/early/2011/02/21/peds.2010-1465.full.pdf An example of the TRACK test is on the third page of the article.

Your doctor might get this information from the child's chart or from you through a friendly chat during your child's doctors visit. However this information is collected, it can be helpful in helping your doctor to understand how well your child's asthma is being controlled. TRACK is a fairly new tool and wasn't included in the Expert Panel's third report.

ATAQ: Asthma Therapy Assessment Questionaire

The asthma therapy assessment questionaire is another quick, simple tool to help your doctor see if your asthma is being well controlled. The ATAQ has versions for pediatrics, adolescents, and adults. The result of any of the tests will help the doctor get an idea of how well the asthma is being controlled.

The ATAQ has three to five multiple choice questions and each response is either a zero or a one. The questions are about the control of your asthma and the final answer will range from zero to four. An answer of one or more says you have less control of your asthma. This information will help your doctor decide what to do next.

Ask your doctor if you could take the ATAQ. You can see what the ATAQ looks like if you go to this site: File.tmp/AdultATAQ.pdf. The information will help both you and your doctor. The more information you have about management of your asthma, the better you'll be able to manage it.

ACQ: Asthma Control Questionaire

The asthma control questionaire was developed in England to help health care providers measure asthma control and the changes in asthma control. The ACQ has seven questions and each question is important. Leaving out any of the questions can make the test inaccurate and unreliable as a tool for evaluating asthma control.

The questions are mostly the same as the other asthma assessment questionaires we've discussed so far: asthma symptoms, activity limitation, and use of quick-relief medicine. An additional issue is followed in the ACQ: airway caliber. Measurement of how well is the airway itself is doing is done by measuring FEV1%(FEV1 and peak flows will be discussed in a later chapter).

The five questions based on symptoms ask about waking at night due to your asthma troubles, waking up in the morning with breathing troubles, how able you are to do the things you usually do and about your shortness of breath and wheezing. The remaining two questions dealing with airway caliber uses questions about your FEV1 and quick-relief medicine use.

In general, if your total is less than one, your asthma is well controlled and totals greater than one says your asthma is not well controlled.

This test has been validated and could be useful to your health care provider to know when your asthma is or isn't being controlled and if there has been any change in the control of your asthma. The asthma control questionaire can be seen here: http://ajrccm.atsjournals.org/content/162/4/1330.full. This is the actual test developed by Elizabeth Juniper.

ACT: Asthma Control Test

The asthma control test is a short, five question test for measuring your asthma control. The standard ACT is for 12 year olds and older but there is a childhood asthma control test (C-ACT) for children four years to eleven years of age. This test measures control by asking questions about your quick-relief medicine use, your nighttime or early morning awakenings, or your shortness of breath, wheezing, or chest tightness. The last question of the five asks how would you grade your degree of control.

The ACT seeks the same goal as the other three assessment tools: to get a good feel of how well your asthma is being controlled. This information will help your health care provider decide what would be the best thing for you. Knowing how well controlled your asthma is can help your doctor decide which medicines you should be taking, how much of it you should be taking and even how often you should be taking it.

You can see what the ACT looks like by visiting http://www.asthma.com/resources/asthma-control-test.html.

Understanding how to use an asthma care plan and being familiar with the purpose of assessment tools can be very important in helping you to keep control of your asthma.

Asthma Medicine Devices and Equipment

Quick-relief medicines and control medicines can be taken in many different ways. Some medicines are better taken in certain ways. Some medicines are inhaled as an aerosol while others are swallowed as a pill. Some are inhaled as a dry powder while others are taken as a shot. Let's consider some of the ways asthma medicines are taken and list a few medicines that are taken in each different way.

Metered Dose Inhaler (MDI)

Quick-relief, controller medicines and combinations of quick-relief and controller medicines can be taken as a metered dose inhaler. This inhaler is a device which delivers a 'metered dose' or specific amount of medicine with each squeeze of the canister and the actuator. Each burst of aerosolized medicine carries a certain dose of medicine to be inhaled. Depending on the medicine, the sometimes included stabilizing agent and the particular inhaler, the specific dose can change if the inhaler is dropped or left lying unused for long periods. The manufacturers instructions should always be followed closely.

Many of the quick-relief medicines can be found in the MDI form. A short list includes: albuterol (Ventolin, Pro-Air, Proventil, Volmax and others), and levalbuterol (Xopenex). A number of controller medicines can also be found at the pharmacy in MDI form. A few controller medicines in MDI form include beclomethasone (Qvar), flunisolide (Aerobid), and fluticasone (Flovent). Some medicines combine quick-relief ingredients with controller ingredients and place them together in one metered dose inhaler. A couple of examples are budesonide and formoterol which are sold as Symbicort and another is fluticasone and salmeterol which is sold as Advair.

All of these inhalers have a limited number of bursts of medicine within them. These devices will sometimes seem to still have medicine in them even after they've run out. Be sure that you know how many puffs of medicine your device started with so you can know when all the medicine is gone. Some of the MDIs have counters on them to help you know when you've run out. Remember that you must keep count of your puffs even if the MDI doesn't have a counter. You can do this by simply making a mark on a sheet of paper each time you express a puff of medicine.

Metered dose inhalers should always be used with spacers. A spacer can be as simple as the cardboard in the center of a toilet paper roll or as complicated as a valved holding chamber. Either is better than spraying the medicine into your mouth from just the inhaler itself. When the particles of medicine are propelled from the inhaler, the bigger particles land on the tongue, roof of the mouth and back of the throat. Without perfectly matching the medicine burst with breathing in, you won't get much of the medicine to go where it's needed; in the lungs. The use of spacers makes perfect timing unnecessary.

Use the following steps to get the best treatment when you're using an MDI.

1. **Shake the inhaler good and hard for several seconds.** This makes sure that the mix of medicine and propellant is perfect to give you the amount of medicine you're supposed to get in each puff.

2. A valved holding chamber is the best type of spacer to use. It doesn't require you to have perfect timing when you squirt the medicine and breathe it in. The medicine can float in the chamber for a second or two while you suck it in. **Place the inhaler in the spacer then place the spacer mouthpiece into your mouth and squirt one puff by pressing down on the top of the inhaler and up on the bottom at the same time.** Make sure that you blow out some air before you do this. You want to make sure to have room in your lungs before you give yourself the medicine.

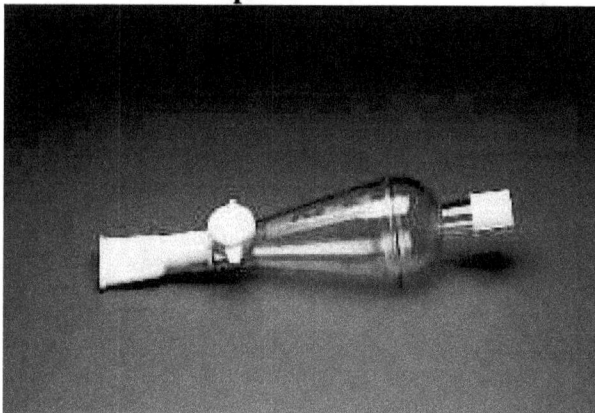

ACE Spacer   **Mouthpiece Aerochamber**

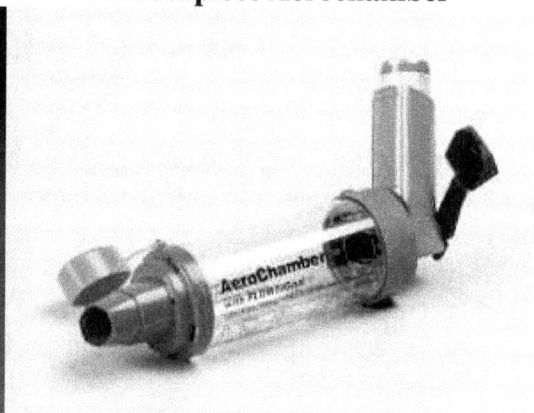

Small Mask Aerochamber

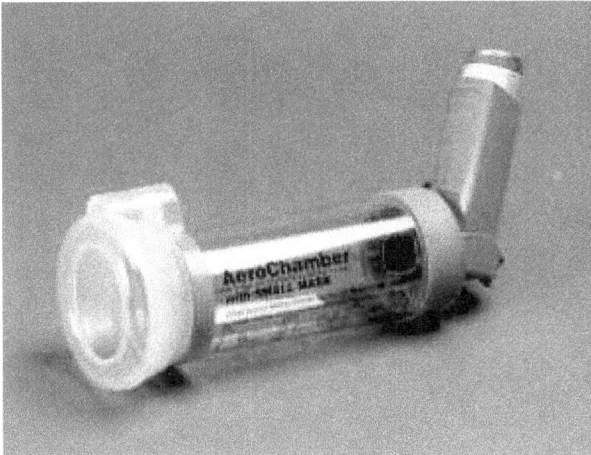

Medium Mask Aerochamber

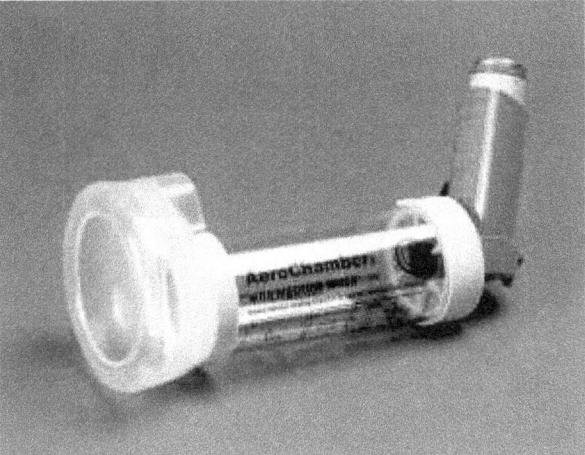

Easivent

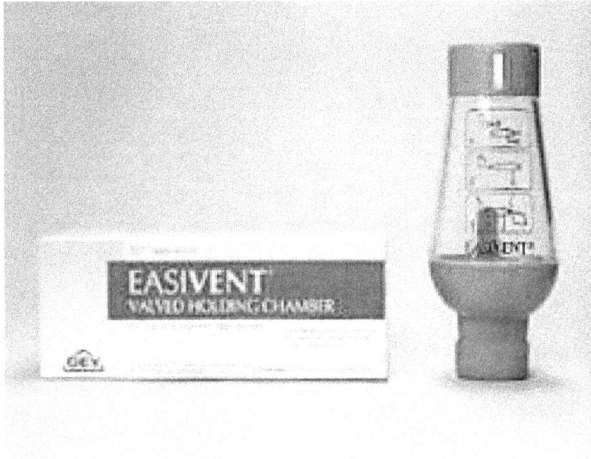

Ellipse

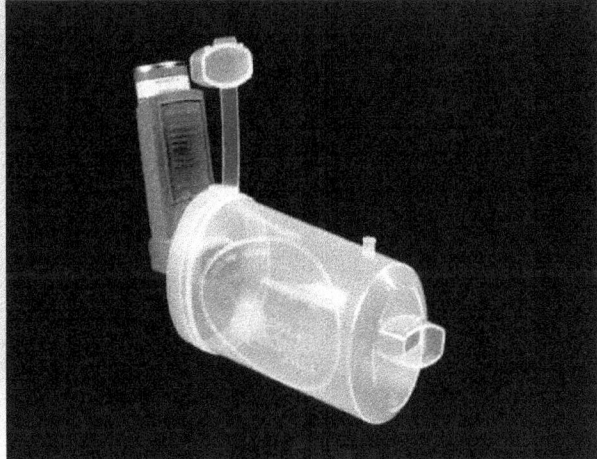

E-Z Spacer

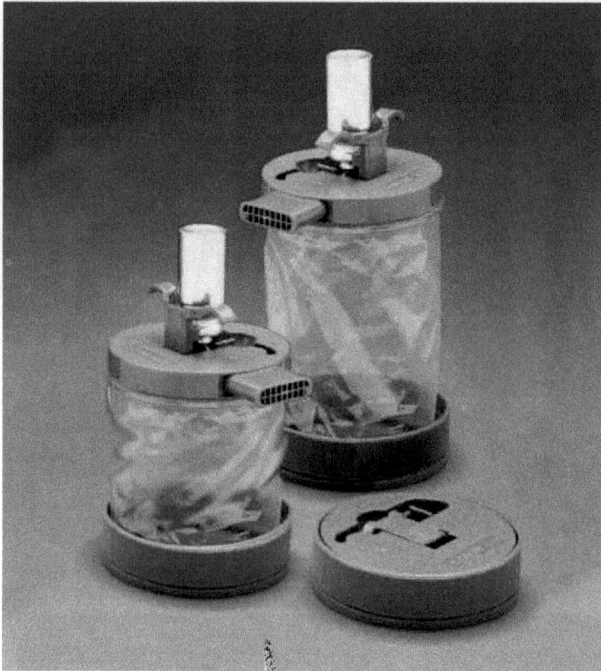

Inspirease

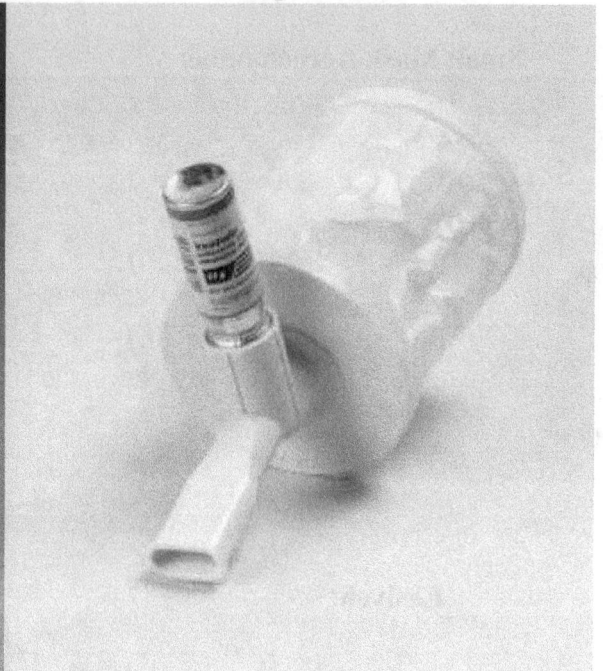

Medispacer

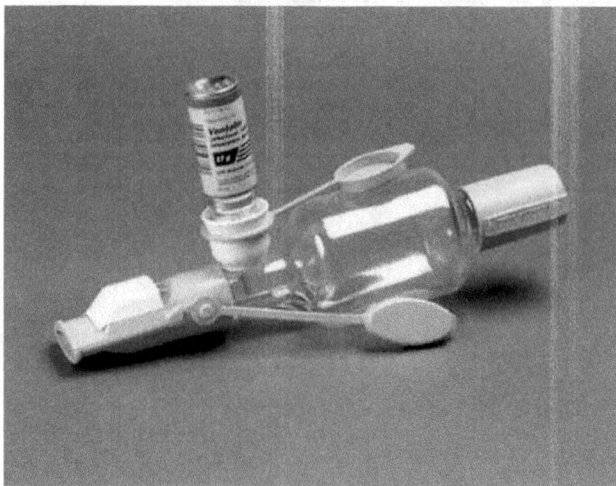

LiteAire

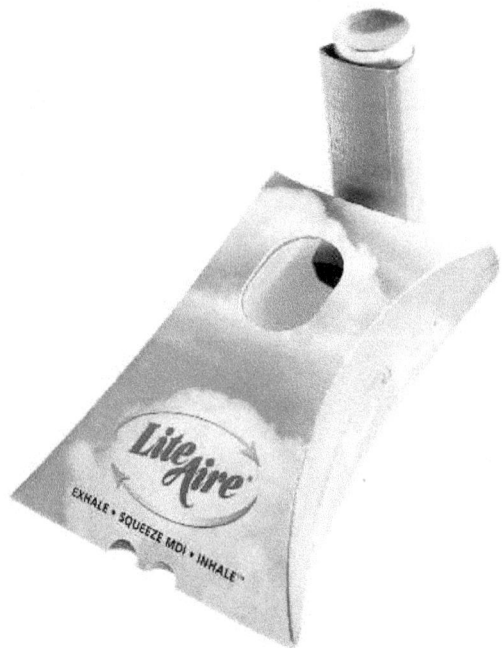

Optichamber   **Nebuhaler**

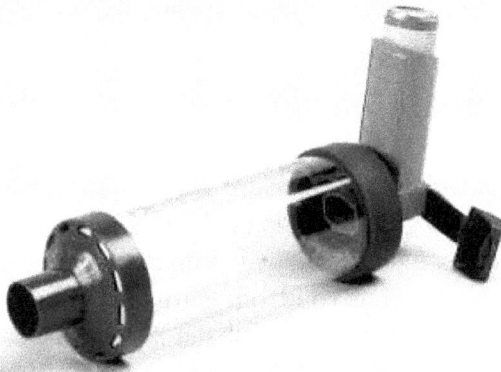

RiteFlo

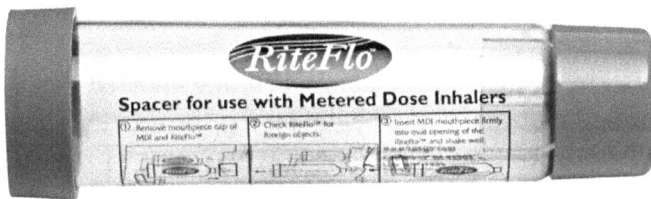

Spacers come in many different types. Some have valves and some don't. Some collapse when you inhale and others don't. Some inhalers will cost more than others. If you can possibly get a spacer of any kind, you'll receive a better treatment than you will without a spacer.

Spacers reduce your side effects by catching the big particles which would bump into your tongue or throat. Your tissues would absorb the medicine and you would have more side effects. Your heart rate would increase and you'd become more jittery if it's quick-relief medicines you're taking. You might get oral thrush or voice changes if it's controllers you're taking.

IMPORTANT: When it's controllers you're taking, remember to rinse you're mouth after each dose. A fungal infection called 'thrush' could develop in your mouth if you don't. If you're using a mask to give the controller to a young child, wash the area of the face which was covered by the mask once the treatment is finished and wash the mask.

3. **Take a slow, deep breath**. Make it slow enough to last over several seconds. The slower and deeper the breath you take, the better treatment you'll get.

4. **You should now hold that breath as long as you can**. Try to hold your breath for 10 seconds. Just slowly count to ten and that should be long enough.

5. **Now you should rest until you feel comfortable and ready for another puff**. This is an important step since you won't be able to hold your breath for very long if you don't rest. Of course you'll repeat these steps until you've given yourself the number of puffs your doctor has prescribed.

There is an excellent reason for each step. Step number one is to make sure you mix the medicine well before you take any. Step number two says to press the top of the inhaler and the bottom of the inhaler (not the bottom of the spacer) at the same time. This is important because some spacers compress a little when squeezed. This might prevent you from getting as good a puff as you would have received if you pressed the top and bottom of the inhaler. Step three says take a slow, deep breath. Fast breaths will cause most of the medicine to go to the back of the throat where it will be swallowed instead of inhaled. Shallow breaths will not allow the medicine to go where the breathing problem is located. Step four says you should hold your breath as long as you can or until a slow count to ten. A long breath hold allows the small particles of medicine to settle out of the air stream you sucked the medicine in on. If you don't hold your breath long, most of the medicine will float out on your next breath since the particles are very small and lightweight. Then of course you should rest because you can't hold your breath long if you don't rest between slow, deep inspirations.

IMPORTANT: Virtually all MDIs will need to be primed before using. Priming an MDI means to throw away a few puffs before using it for the first time. Not all MDIs are primed in the same way. For some it's two puffs and for others it's three or four puffs. Check with your pharmacist and the documents within the medicine package to know how many puffs to waste before you use your brand new MDI canister.

You should clean your spacer about once weekly. This is easily done by filling a bowl with warm clean water. Add a teaspoon of dishwashing liquid and mix it up. Place the spacer in the soapy mixture and allow it to soak for about thirty minutes. Take it out, shake off the excess water and let it air dry without rinsing. The LiteAire spacer (see image above) doesn't require cleaning. It is an inexpensive cardboard spacer and is disposable after one week's use.
The thin soapy mixture will clean the spacer and block the buildup of electrostatic charge within the spacer. The charge buildup occurs in many of the plastic spacer types. Antistatic materials are often used in spacers to resist electrostatic charge buildup. An electrostatic charge can stop some of your medicine from reaching your lungs so weekly soaking of your spacer in a thinly soaped mixture can help you get the dosage your doctor has prescribed.

Dry Powder Inhaler (DPI)

There are many respiratory medicines that are formulated as dry powders. Some quick-relief medicines and some controller medicines are DPIs as are some combination (quick-relief and controller together) medicines. Here is a short list of medicines that can be found in the dry powder inhaler form: Formoterol, Fluticasone, Salmeterol and Fluticasone together, Budesonide, Terbutaline, and Albuterol. Below are a few examples of dry powder inhalers. These images are **curtesy of Michael J. Schumacher** of the University of Arizona.

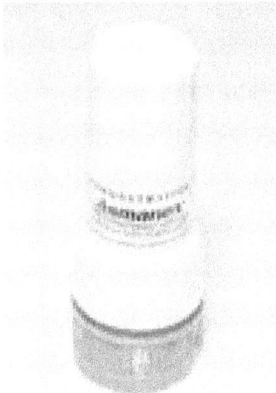

Asmanex   Flovent Diskus   Pulmicort Flexhaler

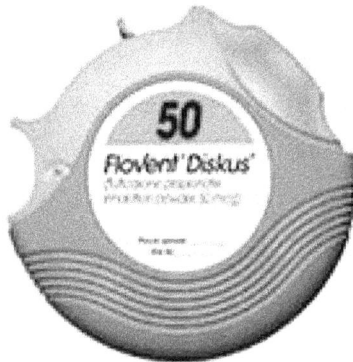

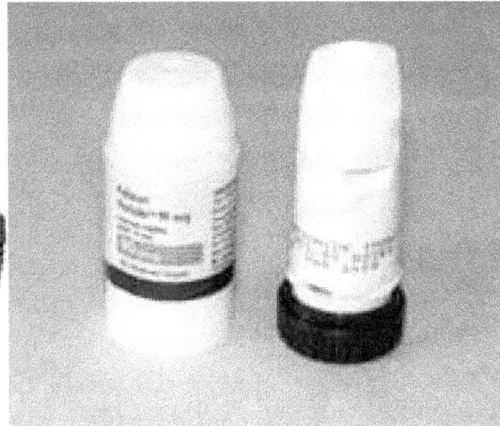

Dry powder inhalers don't use spacers. The device carrying the dry powder is itself the spacer too. So you don't have to concern yourself with spacers if you're using a dry powder inhaler.

You take DPIs just like you would MDIs except that the technique you use is a little different. Small children or the elderly might not be able to use dry powder inhalers because you have to suck the medicine in with a strong, fast breath. The medicine still goes directly to the lungs to provide its benefits. However these devices have major differences from MDIs and it is very important that proper technique is used or you won't be helped by using them.

IMPORTANT: Since it is a dry powder, it must not be allowed to get damp or wet. The medicine will clump up and never leave the inhaler when you suck on it if it becomes damp or wet. You must not store the DPI in a high humidity place and you must never breathe back into the inhaler. Your breath is damp and breathing back into the inhaler will ruin your inhaler and all the medicine within the inhaler will be lost.

The many different devices that are dry powder inhalers require slightly different techniques for the particular device. The general technique listed below isn't specific to any particular device but to the general use of dry powder inhalers as a group.

1. **Turn your face away from the device and blow out all your air.** You want to have an empty lung when you put your mouth on the mouthpiece so that you'll be able to suck in strong and fast.

2. **Place your mouth on the mouthpiece and suck in fast and strong and deep.** You may or may not taste or feel the medicine you've just sucked in but trust that you now have it in your lungs.

3. **Now hold your breath for a slow count of ten seconds.** It is important that you remove the device away from your mouth at the time you start the breath hold. You don't want any air to escape you and get back into the device. After you've

held your breath as long as you can, let it out <u>away</u> from the device and repeat the steps if your prescription calls for more medicine.

How you hold the device or how you get the medicine ready within the device for your big strong inward suck will be slightly different between devices. The common thread between them all will be the three steps above.

Nebulizers

While dry powder inhalers would be hard for a small child or elderly person to use, nebulizers would be easy. Nebulizers make the medicine available to you by using an external source of air flow. A small bore tube is connected from a compressed air source to a small reservoir for the medicine. The air flows into the reservoir at a fast enough rate to break up the medicine into very small breathable particles. The medicine can then be inhaled through a mouthpiece or a mask. A mask is the choice for children five or younger or the aged. A mask is useful for anyone who is unable to form a seal around a mouthpiece and intelligently suck air in through the mouth alone. If unable to do this because of disability, youth or incapacitation, a mask is the best choice.

Nebulizers are used for anticholinergics, steroids, short acting beta agonists and other categories of respiratory medicines.

Below is an image of a nebulizer with medicine reservoir and small bore tube.

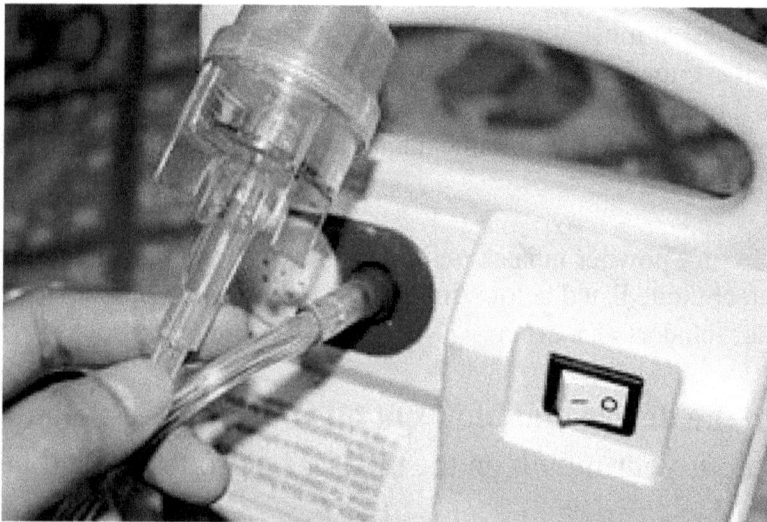

Nebulizer

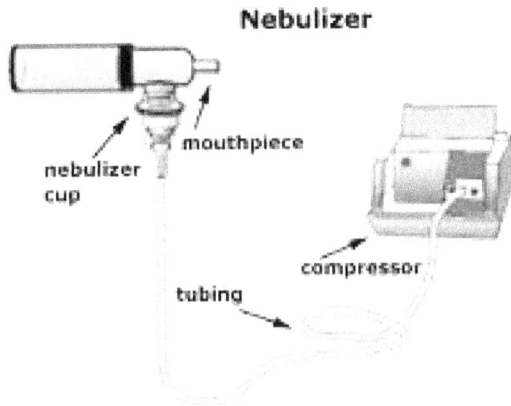

Unlike MDIs or DPIs, nebulizers require electricity to work. You cannot run a nebulizer of the type shown in this picture from your car. However, there are some battery powered nebulizers available now. Check with your pharmacy and doctor about where you can get a nebulizer if your medicine requires one.

Albuterol   Atrovent

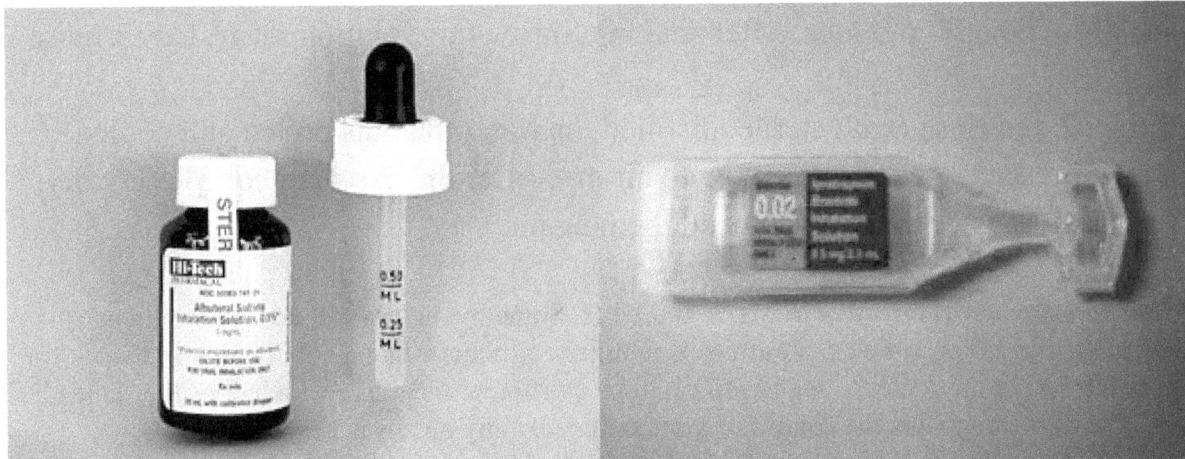

The albuterol and atrovent in this picture can be used in a nebulizer like the one above.

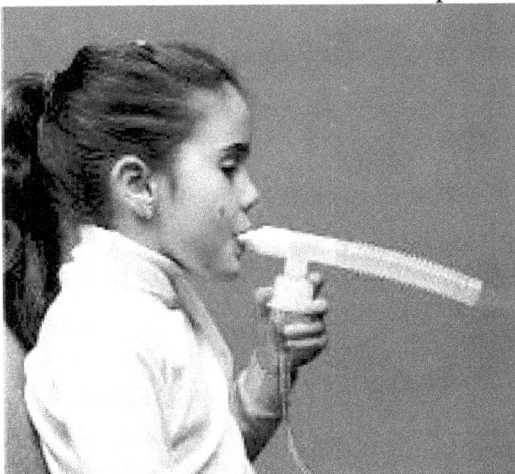

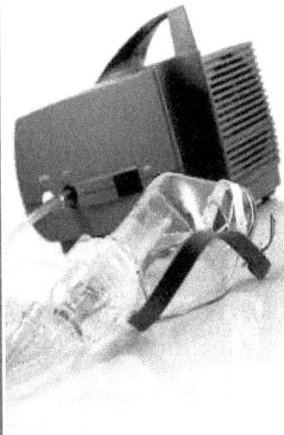

A nebulizer with a mouthpiece and one with a mask

Nebulizers must be cleaned every couple of days to keep it free of germs. It is best to check the cleaning directions given by the manufacturer of the nebulizer. If you don't have that, you can follow these general directions:

1. Wash the nebulizer parts (nebulizer reservoir for the medicine, mouthpiece, and mask) in warm soapy water. The extension tube can be wiped down.
2. Rinse with distilled or sterile water if you have it. If not, you can boil some water for ten or twenty minutes, let it cool and use that to rinse with.
3. Allow the nebulizer machine to blow through the reassembled nebulizer parts for five or ten minutes to help them to dry then take them apart again.
4. Mix one part white vinegar (about 1/2 cup) to three parts distilled or sterile water (about 1 1/2 cups) in a large bowl. Use water that has boiled and cooled if you don't have distilled or sterile water. Place the nebulizer parts in the mixture to soak for about 30 minutes. After soaking, throw this solution away. Don't reuse it.
5. Remove and rinse (with sterile, distilled, or water that has boiled and cooled)
6. Shake off excess water and allow to air dry. After the parts are **completely** dry, seal in ziplock bags until you need them again.

Nebulizers are just as effective as MDIs and DPIs. Some medicines can be found only as nebulizable medicines. If you can't afford a nebulizer or believe that a nebulizer won't work for you, check with your doctor to see if you can take a different medicine which does the same thing. The ultimate goal is the control of your asthma by any means necessary.

Recommended Technique for Various Devices

There are a large number of different devices used to deliver asthma medicines to the lungs. There are almost as many different techniques to use those devices properly.

The sections on MDIs and DPIs had instructions on how to actually take medicine with those devices included in the section. Let's begin this section with some other device types and how to use them to take medicine correctly.

Nebulizers

Using nebulizers is easy.

1. **Open the nebulizer cup and squirt in the medicine.** It might be in a premixed vial or you might have to mix it. Your doctor or pharmacist will tell you how much medicine to add.

2. **Connect the small bore tubing to the bottom of the nebulizer cup and to the source of the compressed air (usually an electric nebulizing device)**

3. **Turn on your nebulizing device.** The flow rate is probably preset.

4. As the medicine turns to misty, aerosolized particles, **take slow deep breaths of the medicine.** If you breath normally for four or five breaths then let your next breath be a slow deep breath, you'll be taking your medicine very effectively without getting tired.

5. **Continue taking the medicine in this way until the mist stops coming out.** Tap the device to make sure the medicine has finished before you turn off the air compressor.

Twisthalers

Twisthalers are easy devices to use. These differ from some of the other devices in that twisthalers only release the medicine when you suck in. There is no button to press and the medicine doesn't just come out when air is flowed through it.

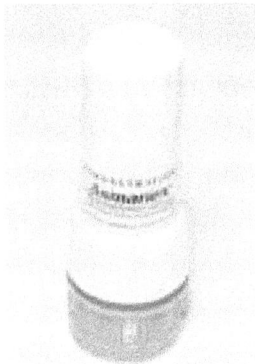

This image is **curtesy of Michael J. Schumacher** of the University of Arizona.

Mometasone Furoate (Asmanex) is one medicine which uses this type of dispenser. Asmanex is a dry powder inhaler so all the important information you remember from the previous section on DPIs applies to using this twisthaler device.

1. **Hold the twisthaler upright with the pink or grey portion facing down toward the floor and the white portion facing up toward the ceiling.** *Don't* shake the device to get it ready.

2. **Twist the top to the left (counterclockwise) to remove it.** By twisting it, you open and load a dose of medicine within the device. The indented portion of the twisthaler will line up with the counter. The counter, which tells how much medicine remains within the twisthaler, is reduced by one number. If the counter read sixty before you twist the top, it will read 59 after you twist the top.

3. **Now turn your face away from the twisthaler and breathe out all your air.** This is important because you want to be able to suck in fast and deeply when you start taking your dose.

4. **Hold the twisthaler horizontally (sideways), put the mouthpiece into your mouth and seal your mouth tightly around the mouthpiece. Take a fast, deep breath out of the twisthaler.**

5. **Hold your breath as long as you can or for 10 seconds.** Move the twisthaler away from your mouth right after you suck medicine out of it and before you start breath holding. Remember that dry powder inhalers must remain dry inside so you must be very careful when your mouth is near it that you don't accidentally allow breath to enter the device. You'll clump up and lose your medicine if you breathe back into the twisthaler.

6. **Now just dry the mouthpiece with a clean dry cloth or tissue and replace the cover. Turn the cover to the right (clockwise) to close.** You'll hear two clicks and the arrow-shaped indention will line up with the counter when it has been closed correctly. Repeat these steps for each dose your doctor or pharmacist has told you to take.

7. **Remember to rinse your mouth with water and spit after your final dose.** Asmanex is a steroid and might cause fungus to grow in your mouth if you don't remember to rinse and spit after using it.

That's it. Easy right? The important thing to remember is don't breathe into it. Breathing just a little into the twisthaler will ruin all the remaining medicine so make sure that you don't let that happen.

Rotahalers

   Below are a few images of a rotahaler. Both quick-relief and controller medicines can be found as a rotahaler. One image below shows the rotahaler as a quick-relief medicine; Ventolin. Another shows the rotahaler with a capsule inserted.

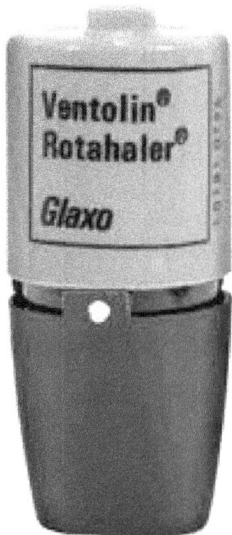

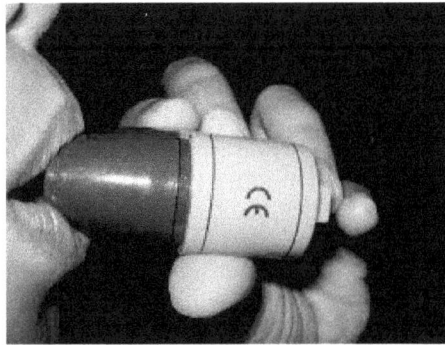

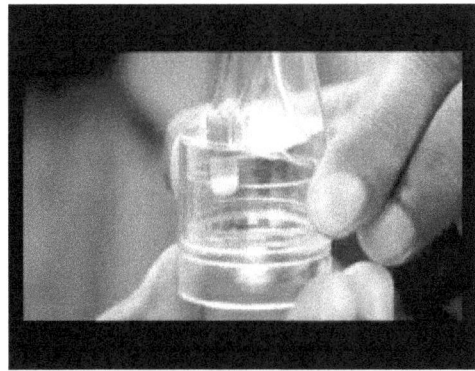

   The technique of using the rotahaler is also easy. Rotahalers are dry powder inhalers so all the rules of using dry powder inhalers (DPIs) apply to the rotahaler. The rotahaler device, however, has its own specific directions. They are two-piece devices which can be separated and cleaned. This is one of the few dry powder devices like this. Since it dispenses one capsule at a time, it becomes empty after each dose. Because of this it can be cleaned.
   Ventolin rotahalers can no longer be found in the United States but there are still several respiratory medicines that use this type of dry powder inhaler. Symbicort, Advair, and Pulmicort are three medicines that can still be found to use the rotahaler.
   Here are general directions for using the rotahaler. If your doctor or pharmacist has directed you to follow different directions for a specific medicine, do as your health care provider or pharmacist directs.

1. Remove the rotahaler from its container. **Hold it upright and rotate the lower half in either direction**. The upper half is dark and is the mouthpiece. The lower half is light and is the part you rotate.
2. **Get a rotatab and insert it into the hole in the lighter colored end.** The capsule is two-toned also. **The lighter end of the capsule should be the first to go into the hole. Push it in until the whole capsule is inserted and your**

finger is flush with the hole. It should look like the image above when the capsule has been properly inserted.

3. **Rotate the bottom of the rotahaler until it contacts the capsule and breaks it.** Powder will fall into the lower half along with the clear half of the capsule.

4. **Turn your face away from the rotahaler and blow out all your air.** You want to be able to suck in a fast, deep breath when you insert the mouthpiece into your mouth.

5. **Place the mouthpiece into your mouth and suck a fast, deep breath into your lungs.** Remove the rotahaler from your mouth while you hold your breath.

6. **Hold your breath for 10 seconds or as long as you can.** Repeat these steps until you've taken all medicine as the doctor has prescribed.

7. You should clean your rotahaler twice a month. Remove the loose capsule from the lower part of the rotahaler and from the capsule hole. **Wash out the rotahaler with warm soapy water and rinse well. Dry it completely before putting it up for safe keeping. It must be completely dry before storing.**

Using a rotahaler is easy and by following these directions you'll be taking your medicine in the recommended way.

Diskus

Below are two images of a diskus. The blue one is an Advair diskus which combines a steroid with a long acting beta agonist. The orange one is a steroid diskus.

There are a number of respiratory medicines that use the diskus. The diskus is another dry powder inhaler device. Dry powder inhalers (DPIs) are breath activated which means you get the medicine when you suck a deep breath from the mouthpiece of the device. These devices have a convenient dose counter so that you can know when you've run out of medicine. The counter tells you how much medicine remains. Each time you take a dose, the counter shows that the number remaining has gone down by one.

Notice the image below with the parts of the diskus labeled.

Some general instructions for diskus use follows.

Outer Case

Dose Indicator

50
Flovent Diskus

Mouthpiece

Thumbgrip

Lever

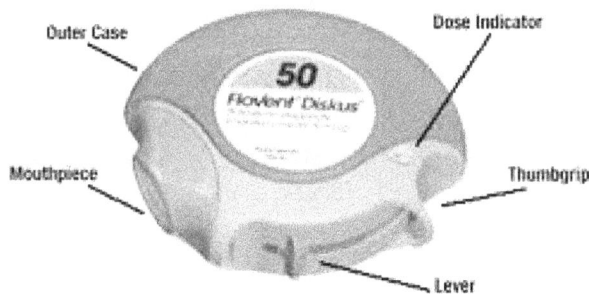

1. **Hold the diskus in your hand. With your other hand, slide the thumbgrip around until you hear a click.** This action brings the mouthpiece into view.

2. **Slide the lever all the way down until you hear a click.** This action loads your dose of medicine.

3. Hold the diskus level (horizontally), **turn your face away from the diskus and blow out all your air.** You want to be able to suck in a fast, deep breath when you take your dose.

4. **Put the mouthpiece into your mouth and suck in a fast, deep breath.** Fill your lungs from the diskus in that one breath.

5. **Remove the diskus from your mouth and hold your breath.** Try to hold your breath for 10 seconds but do hold it as long as you can.

6. **Breathe out and rest. Be sure not to breathe out toward the diskus.** It is important that no breath gets back into the diskus or the breath will ruin your dry powder.

7. **Close the device by pushing the thumbgrip back to where it started out.** If you have another dose to take, repeat the steps above. When you've taken the last dose, wipe the mouthpiece with a clean cloth and close the diskus by sliding the thumbgrip to it's starting place.

IMPORTANT: Remember to rinse your mouth and spit after each treatment if there is a steroid in the diskus. If you're unsure if a steroid is in it, rinse and spit until you can find out if there is or not. You could develop thrush in your mouth if you forget to rinse and spit after your dose. ***Don't wash the diskus. The diskus must always remain dry.***

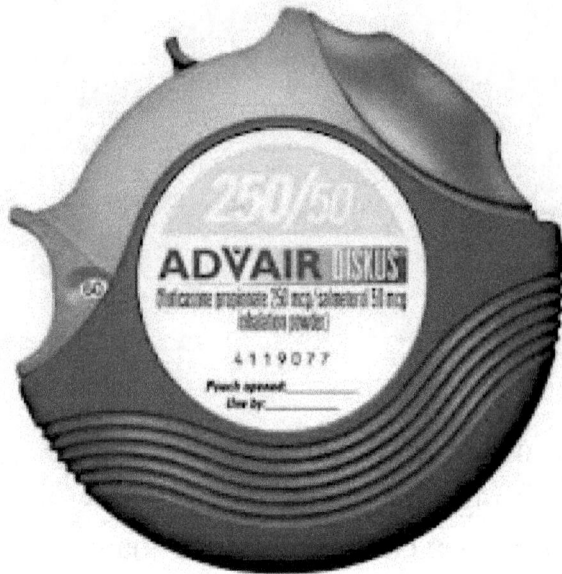

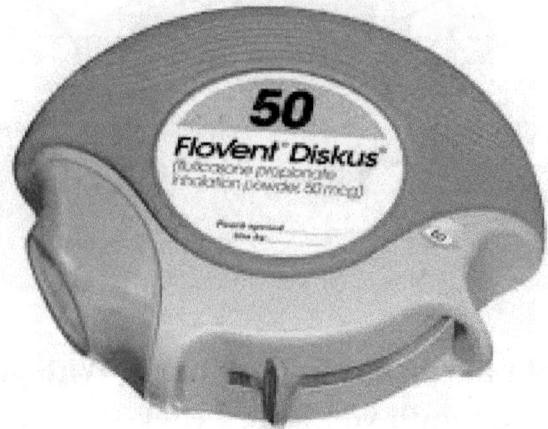

Turbohalers

Mouthpiece with spiral shaped channels
Extra air inlets
Inhalation channel
One metered dose
Rotating dosing disk
Drug reservoir
Air inlet
Turning grip
Scrapers
Drying agent

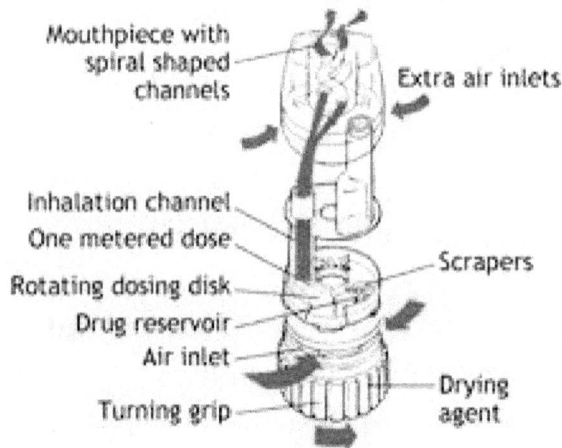

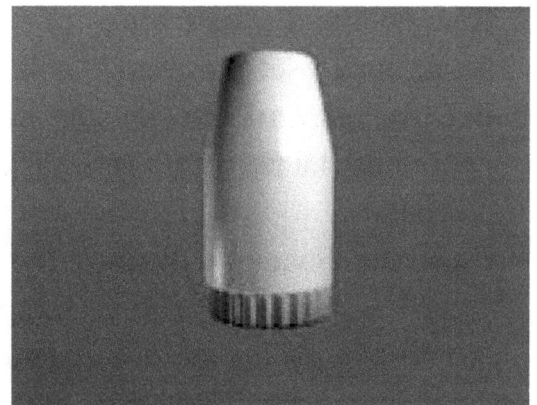

Turbutaline and Budesonide are two medicines that can be found as turbohalers (sometimes spelled turbuhalers). Turbutaline is a bronchodilator and budesonide is a steroid. You will usually find the medicine in a turbohaler to be a steroid.

Using the turbohaler is as easy as using any of the other dry powder devices. The same important reminders apply to the turbohaler as to the other devices. Remember to keep moisture away from the turbohaler since it is a dry powder device. If moisture gets inside with the dry powder, the powder will no longer be dry and you won't be able to get the medicine out.

The turbohaler looks like the image on the above right. The bottom portion is the part you turn to load your dose. Once loaded, you should never turn the device upside down or you could lose medicine. You don't need to shake your inhaler and be careful not to drop it.

Most turbohalers will have a counter which will tell you just how many doses you have. Those turbohalers without counters will show a red bar at the top of the counter window when you have 20 doses left. When your inhaler is empty, the red bar will be at the bottom of the counter window. You should keep a written record to accurately keep up with the number of doses you have remaining. Your turbohaler might feel like or sound like it has medicine in it when it doesn't so your record of the actual number of doses will be very helpful.

You should follow the directions given to you when you buy the turbohaler. Ask your pharmacist or doctor any questions you might have about how to use or care for your specific device. Below are general directions on how to use a turbohaler.

1. **Remove the cap**
2. **Hold the turbohaler upright (the colored base should be toward the floor) and turn the base as far as you can in one direction then back the other way until you hear a 'click.'** The click is the sound of your dose being loaded.
3. **Turn your face away from the device and blow out all your air.** You want to be able to suck in a fast, deep breath when you put it into your mouth. You turn your face away from the turbohaler to make sure that you don't get any moisture into the device.
4. **Place the mouthpiece into your mouth between your teeth and form a tight seal with your lips.** Tilt your head slightly back.
5. **Now suck in a fast, deep breath. Remove the turbohaler from your mouth and hold your breath for a slow count to 10 or as long as you can.**
6. Clean the mouthpiece after each use with a dry tissue to remove mouth moisture.

IMPORTANT: It is always important to avoid breathing into a dry powder inhaler device. If it is a steroid that you're taking, remember to rinse your mouth and spit. You could get a fungal infection in the mouth if you forget to rinse.

Using a turbohaler is easy. If you decide it is not something you can do, ask your doctor for a different medicine that does the same thing but comes in a form you feel more comfortable with. The goal is the control of your asthma and you must take your medicine as the doctor orders it to meet that goal.

Accuhalers

An accuhaler is just another name for a diskus. Look at the section on diskus to see how to use and care for an accuhaler.

Autohalers

You can think of autohalers as MDIs that are breath activated and that don't use spacers.

The breath activated MDI or autohaler, looks somewhat different than your regular MDI. Notice the images below of autohalers. The common thing about them all is the lever that sticks out. This lever is raised before you take your deep breath.

The breath activated MDI, which can be a short acting beta agonist (Maxair) or a steroid controller (Qvar), doesn't use a spacer. The autohaler is not a dry powder so you should shake it before you use it. You should place the mouthpiece into your mouth then take a fast deep breath. The instructions for proper technique would be included in the package when you buy it. However, I've included the steps for your convenience.

Remember, if there is a steroid in the autohaler, rinse your mouth and spit after you've taken your dose.

To use an autohaler, follow these steps:

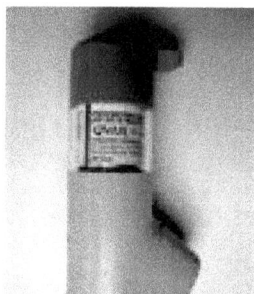

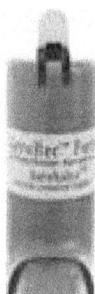

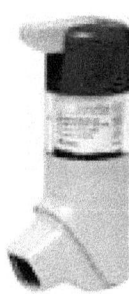

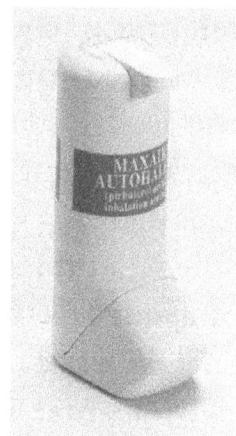

1. **Remove the mouthpiece cover. Hold the inhaler upright. Raise the lever until it snaps into place.**
2. **Shake gently several times.** Hold the inhaler around the middle, making sure to not block the air vents.
3. **Blow out all your air before putting the Autohaler to your lips.** You want to be able to suck in fast and deep when you start.
4. **Place the mouthpiece between your lips and seal your lips around the mouthpiece. Suck in fast and deeply through the mouthpiece.** You will hear a "click" and you'll feel something when the medicine releases. Do NOT stop inhaling until you can't take in any more air.
5. **Hold your breath for 10 seconds, then exhale slowly.** Continue to hold the inhaler upright while lowering the lever.

Notice that the main difference in using the autohaler and other MDIs is how fast you suck the medicine in. Fast for the autohaler and slow for regular MDIs. There is no button to press to make the medicine come out with an autohaler. The medicine comes out only when you suck it out with a deep strong breath and you must have a good seal on the mouthpiece.

As you can see there are a number of types of inhalers for asthma. All of them can be effective if used properly. None of them will be effective if you don't follow the directions for their use. If you've received a prescription for a medicine which uses an inhaler type that you're not comfortable with, ask your doctor to please find you a different medicine. Controller and quick-relief medicines come in many different forms and the chances are great that you can have almost any inhaler form you want to use. Proper use of your inhaler is one important key to controlling your asthma.

Peak Flows and Forced Expired Volumes

Asthma is described as an obstructive lung disease. 'Obstructive' means that your breath is easier to get in than it is to get out. Researchers have long known how to test an asthmatic's ability to breath out and to measure how 'obstructive' their asthma is. When you're having an asthma attack, it is harder to get air out. The bronchoconstriction, airway swelling and increased secretions create more airway obstruction and it takes longer for the air to get out of the lung.

A peak flow meter is a device that measures how much air you can blow out of your lung in one big blast of air. When you're having an attack you can't blow out as much air in one big blast as you can when you're not having an attack.

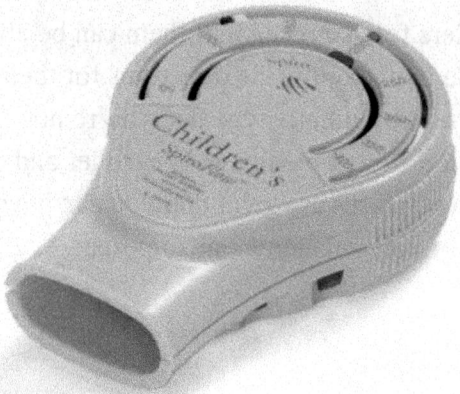

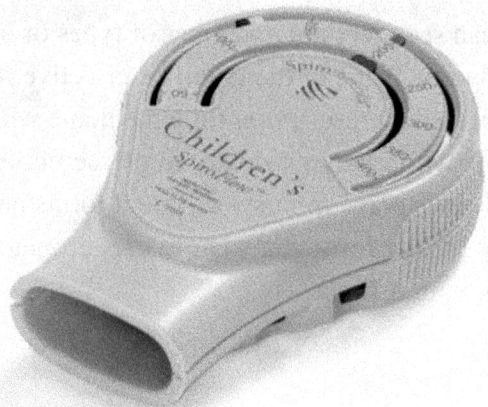

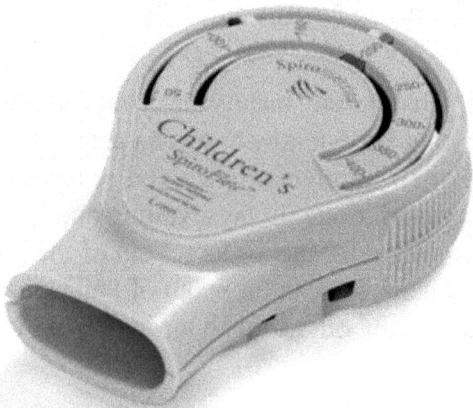

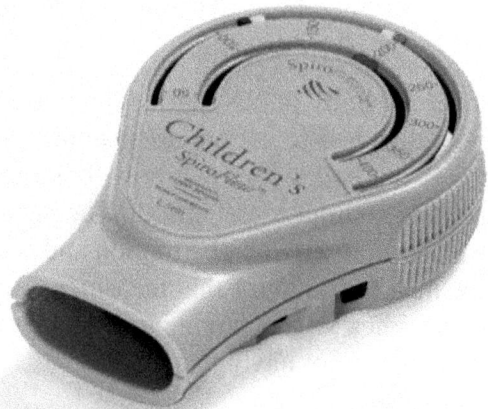

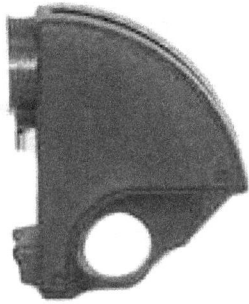

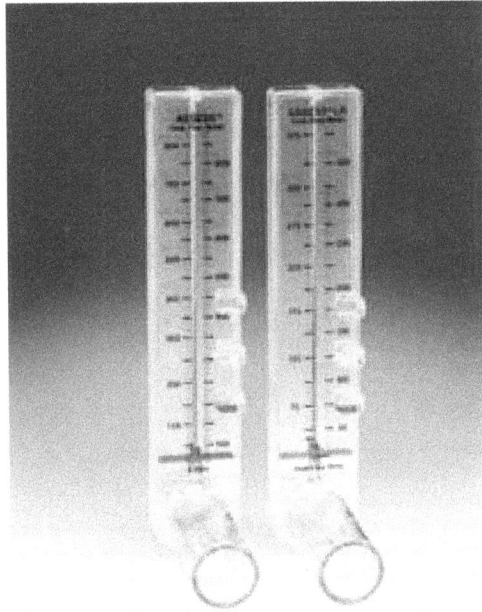

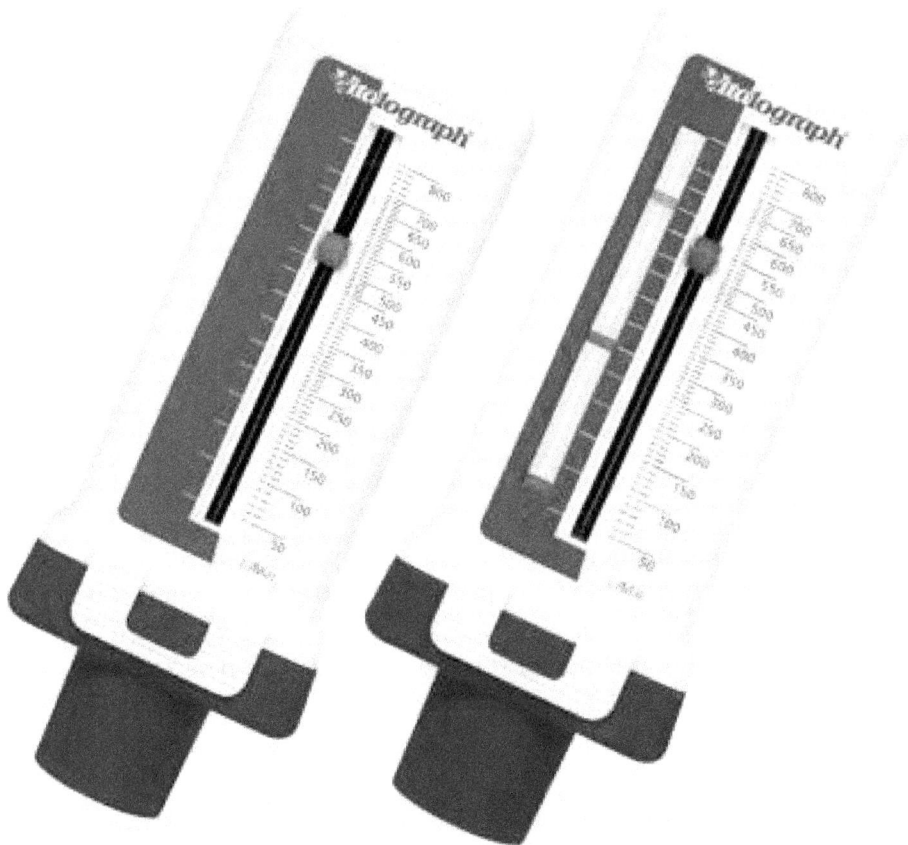

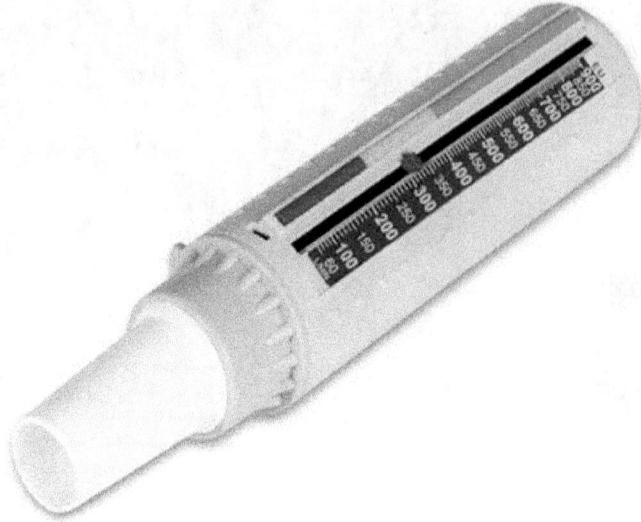

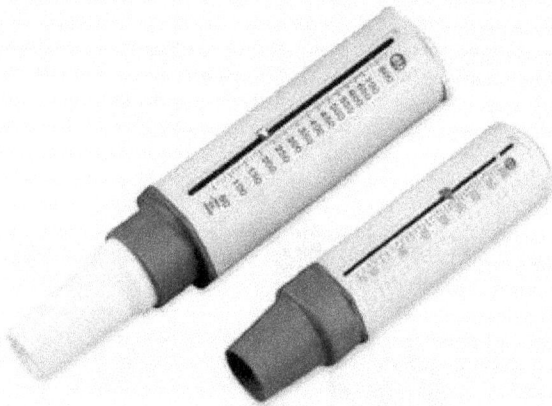

These are images of some of the many types of devices known as peak flow meters. They are all able to measure how much air you can blow out in one big blast of air. When you're doing well, you can blow out more air than when your asthma is bothering you. Even when you think that you're doing well but your airways are already starting to close up, a peak flow meter will still record that less air came out than did when you were at your best. This is why peak flow meters are so valuable. Peak flow meters know when you're starting to do bad sometimes even before you know it.

The Expert Panel suggests that you should use a peak flow meter if asthma attacks often sneak up on you or if your attacks can get pretty bad. As long as you're five or six years old or older and can take in a deep breath and blow it forcefully through the peak flow meter, you can do a peak flow.

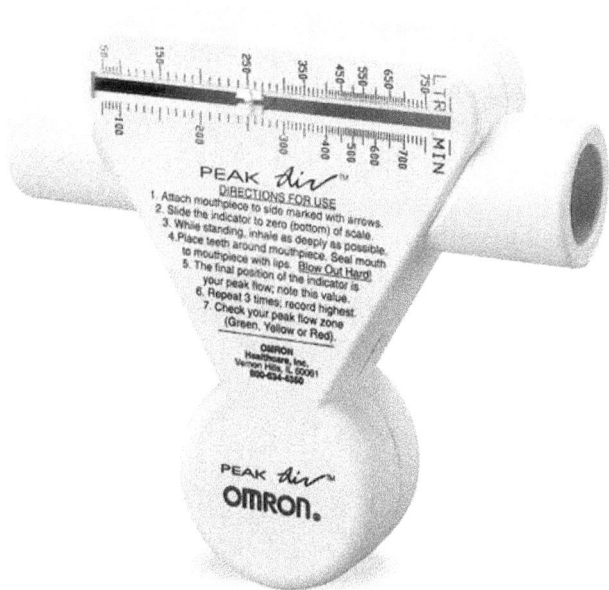

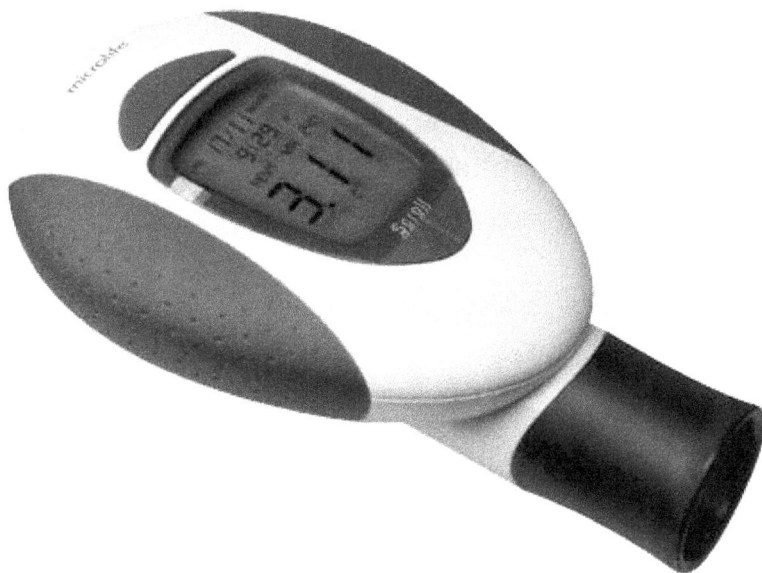

On some of the flow meters you'll notice the colors green, yellow, and red. These colors will match the colors on the action plans. Green is the range where you're doing good. This range is set at 80% or better of the best that you can do. Yellow is the caution color. You're starting to do bad so be watchful. Yellow ranges from 50% of your best to 80% of your best. Red is the color that says you're doing bad right now. Do something quick. Red is set below 50%. If you can blow out only half of what you should be able to blow out then you're in trouble and need to get to an emergency department right now.

How much you can blow out in a single big blast depends on several things. Not only does it depend on how well your asthma is doing, it also depends on your gender (whether you're a boy, girl, man, or woman). It depends on how tall you are (tall people can usually blow out more than short people). How much you can blow out of your lungs in one hugh blast of air even depends on how old you are.

Look at the peak flow scale below. The side of the scale with numbers ranging from 300 (bottom left corner) to 680 (top left corner) are the performance numbers. This is how much air is blown out measured in liters per minute. Notice the arching line for the Men on that scale. The highest point on that line is for taller and younger men. The same for the arching line for the Women.

The technique for doing a peak flow is easy.

1. **Stand up straight.** You can sit upright but standing will usually give you a larger peak flow.
2. **Take a really big breath and prepare to blow it through your peak flow meter.**
3. **Put the peak flow meter mouthpiece in your mouth and blow that air out as fast and forcefully as you can.** Look at the numbers on your flowmeter and see how well you did.
4. Remove it from your mouth and rest briefly so you can do it again. **You should do it three times and keep the best (highest) value.**

You can use that technique with any of the peak flowmeters.

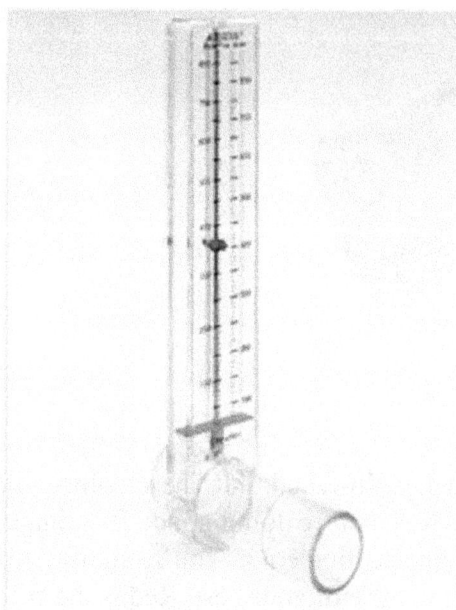

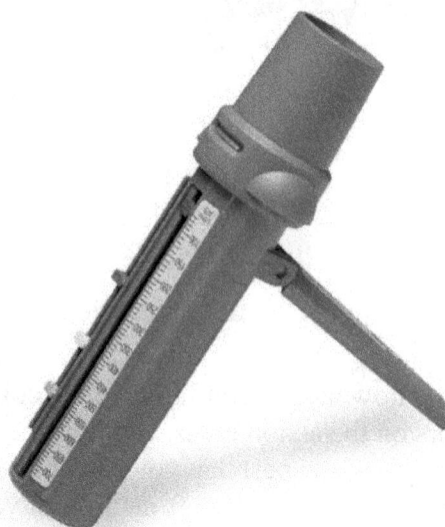

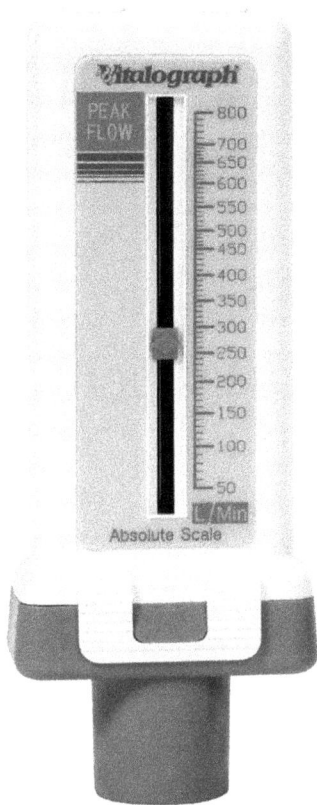

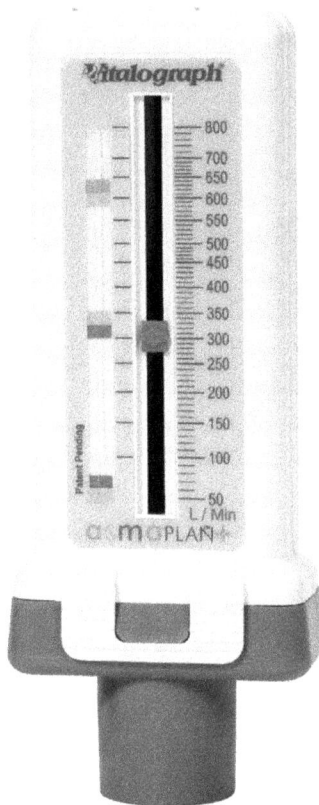

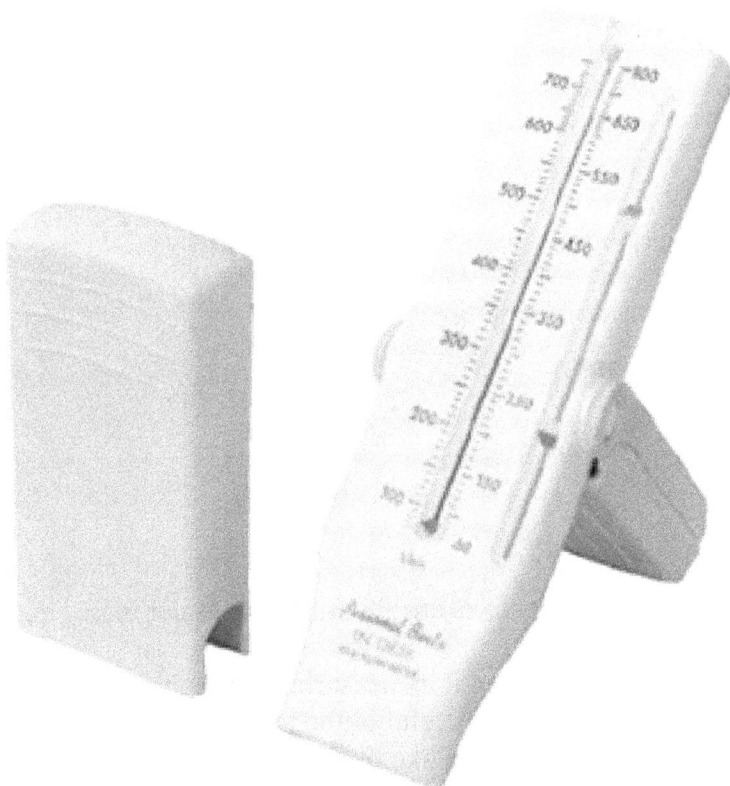

Normal values for peak expiratory flow (PEF)
EN 13826 or EU scale

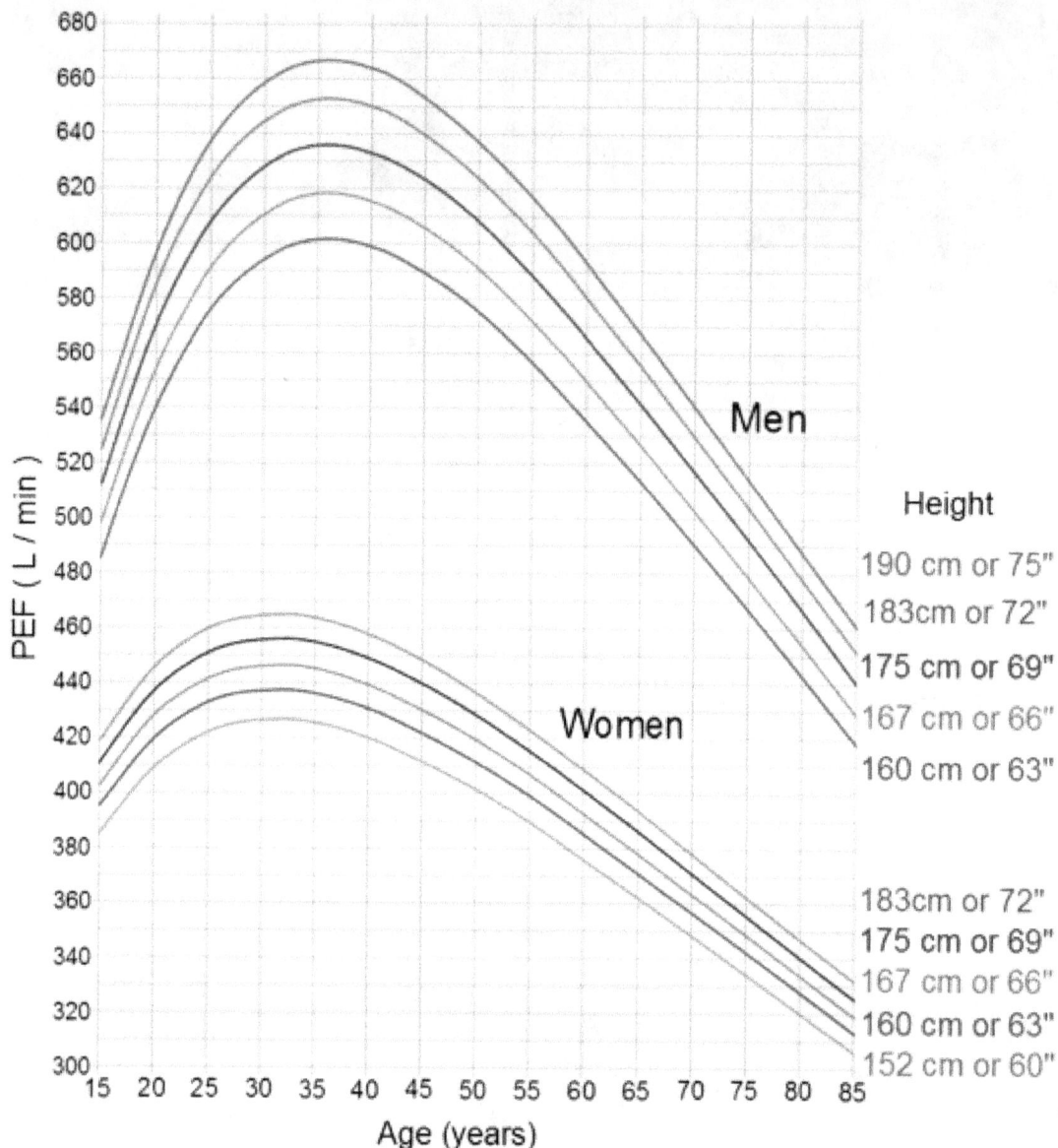

Now that you have a good idea of what flowmeters are about, let's consider forced expired volumes.

Flowmeters and forced expired volumes are helpful in measuring how 'obstructive' your airways are. Forced expired volumes are the more helpful of the two since there are so many types of flowmeters and so much difference in scales like the one above. FEVs (forced expired volumes) measure how much air is blown out as does the flowmeter but FEVs also measure how much time it takes to blow it out. This additional information FEVs give and the weaknesses of the flowmeters make forced expired volumes the doctor's preferred tool when diagnosing asthma. Flowmeters are useful when keeping up with how well your asthma is doing but forced expired volumes are even more useful when figuring out if you have asthma or not.

As we discussed earlier, it takes longer to blow air out of a more obstructed airway than a less obstructed airway. The measurements of efforts to blow air out of obstructed airways have been done so many times that we now know about how long it should take for most of the air to get out. Along with measuring how long it takes for air to be blown out we've learned to measure lung volumes too. Questions like 'How much air is left in your lungs when you think you've blown all of it out?', and 'How much air do your lungs hold when you've sucked in all the air you can?' have been answered. These questions and hundreds of other questions like these about lung volumes, air flow rates, and timed forced expired volumes have been answered.

The study of all these volumes, rates and their relationships to each other along with numerous other types of lung function measurements is called pulmonary functions. It is through pulmonary functions that obstructed airways are better understood. Now when you go to the pulmonary function laboratory, the technician who is practiced in understanding these lung rate and volume relationships can recognize lungs which are most likely asthmatic.

One technique which has been chosen as most useful in helping to tell when a person has asthma is the forced expired volume maneuver. You are asked to blow out all of your air as fast as you can. How much you're able to blow out in a preset time is noted and is compared to what others similar to you (age, gender, etc.) are able to blow out. If the volume you blow out over the same preset time is less than others like you, your airways can be recognized as more obstructed than their airways. The preset time which has been chosen as the most helpful is 1 second. The maneuver is the forced expired volume in 1 second. It's called FEV1 for short.

These pulmonary function tests are good for diagnosing asthma and for keeping up with the condition of asthma. If your doctor tells you that your PFTs (pulmonary function tests) are good, he's really saying that your lungs are generally less obstructed. Air can flow in and out more easily. That tells you that you must be taking your medicines right or that you're avoiding triggers well.

An FEV1 can be measured before you take quick-relief medicine and after you take it. How your airway responds to the medicine gives your doctor important information about your lungs. When you can get more air out in 1 second than you could before, that means your asthma is doing better.

You should keep an ongoing relationship with the pulmonary function laboratory. If you have significant trouble with your asthma you should take a pulmonary function test. Information provided to your doctor by such a test can help your doctor make the best decisions about your care.

Miscellaneous Concerns

Pregnancy

If you have an asthmatic flare-up while you're pregnant, remember that it is worse to have out-of-control asthma than it is to take medicines which might get to the fetus. Asthma that leaves the mother in distress can cause preeclampsia (high blood pressure and increased protein in the urine), low birth weight in the infant, and could even cause the baby to die before it's born.

Making sure that your lungs can maintain the level of oxygen needed to support you and your unborn child means continuing to take your asthma medicines as prescribed.

Each time you report to your doctor for your prenatal visit, get your asthma checked out too. If you find that you need a quick-relief medicine, the Expert Panel recommends albuterol. There is a great deal of information available on albuterol and how safe it is for pregnant asthmatics. If you require a controller during the time you're pregnant, budesonide is the steroid recommended by the Expert Panel. Other steroids are probably just fine but budesonide has the most information available on its use in pregnant mothers.

The important point for you to remember is that you're better off taking your medicines than suffering through chest tightness and difficulty breathing. If you can breath easily you're supplying enough oxygen for yourself and your unborn baby. Your infant could live to thank you for taking your medicine.

Surgery

Surgery carries with it a number of risks to an asthmatic. Even before the scalpel touches you, you have to be sedated and could be allergic to some of the sedating medicines. Latex is seldom used in gloves anymore but if you have an allergy to it, contact with it in any form would be troublesome. Intubation is when the breathing tube is placed in your windpipe to breath for you during your surgery. Intubation has been known to cause airways to tighten up. Sometimes smaller airways completely collapse during the time when your breathing is in the hands of a machine.

It is important that your asthma is behaving at its best if you must have surgery. Don't leave this to your asthma doctor. You take control and make sure that you're taking your medicines properly and that your asthma is well controlled. You should get an appointment to the pulmonary function laboratory to see that everything is as it should be. If the pulmonary functions technician finds something amiss, be sure to tell your doctor right away so that it can be improved before surgery.

Surgery is serious business and even more serious if you have asthma. Make sure that your asthma is in the best possible shape before surgery.

Exercise Induced Bronchospasm (EIB)

This long expression is really quite simple. It is simply talking about how exercise or an increased level of activity can cause your asthma to flare up. When you notice that running to catch the bus or bringing in the groceries can cause you to have trouble breathing, you might be dealing with EIB.

As the name says, exercise causes your asthma to flare up. Bronchospasm is when your airways shrink down a little. It happens when the muscles around your airway tightens up. Usually this happens while some other things are happening too. Like the airway is already inflamed and swollen and possibly filled with secretions. When all of this is going on, a little extra activity like running can make it all very noticeable to you.

Bronchospasm

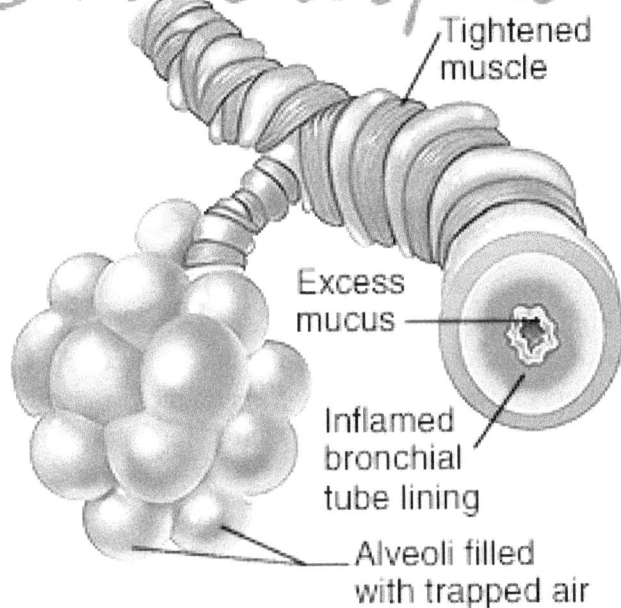

Tightened muscle

Excess mucus

Inflamed bronchial tube lining

Alveoli filled with trapped air

Exercise Induced Bronchospasm can be helped by taking a little albuterol (or other quick-relief medicine) when that happens. You can often prevent the trouble by taking a quick-relief medicine even before the exercise causes the flareup. If you know that EIB is sometimes a problem for you, you should be prepared with a quick-relief medicine to prevent those attacks. A short acting beta agonist (albuterol) or nedocromil (Tilade) would be helpful to you if taken before becoming more active or exercising.

For example, you have to walk up two flights of stairs in your apartment building carrying groceries. Before you even leave the store you could take a few puffs of your medicine so that by the time you get home, your lungs are ready for the challenge.

Sometimes it might be cold air that causes you to have bronchospasm. In that case you should wear a scarf over your mouth and nose so that the cold air won't cause you to have breathing trouble.

As always you should take your control medicines regularly. You'll be able to control your asthma better by regularly taking the medicines your doctor has prescribed. You'll have less trouble with EIB if your airway inflammation is minimal or absent.

Cough Variant Asthma

Asthma that only causes you to cough but not wheeze or even have very much shortness of breath is called cough variant asthma. The coughing can come upon you at any time, day or night. The interesting thing is it doesn't look like asthma because you won't be wheezing. The cough can be caused by exercise like EIB or cold weather. If you have this type of asthma, getting around triggers will increase the coughing.

There are certain medicines that asthmatics should be aware of. These medicines called beta blockers are generally used for the treatment of the heart. Some beta blockers are used in eye drops for the treatment of glaucoma (increased fluid pressure in the eye). If you're taking a beta blocker for some reason and you develop a cough, consider the possibility that it's cough variant asthma and tell your doctor.

Treatment for cough variant asthma is the same as for regular asthma. A short acting beta agonist will cause the coughing to stop if it is really cough variant asthma. Coughing could be from a number of things like post nasal drip or a viral infection. If your coughing is really asthma, medicines taken for asthma will treat cough variant asthma as well.

This variation of regular asthma is something that is fairly often seen and treated. Don't be alarmed if your doctor tells you that you have it. Just continue treating your asthma as you always have. Stick with your regular controllers and keep quick-relief medicines on hand just in case you need them. Remember that cough variant asthma responds well to regular asthma medicine.

Medicines Potentially Harmful to Asthmatics

Beta Blockers

Beta blockers are medicines that block the beta receptors in the body. In the lungs there are beta receptors. There are also beta receptors in the heart. When you take a beta blocker medicine, you block the normal action of the beta receptors in both the heart and lung and where ever else the beta receptor might be.

Blockade of the
Beta$_1$ Receptor Blockers

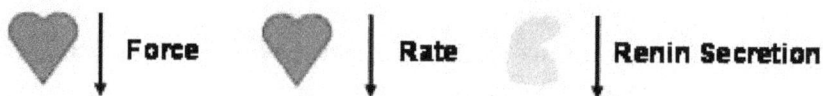

Force   Rate   Renin Secretion

Blockade of the
Beta$_2$ Receptor Blockers

Airway Rresistance   Vascular Resistance

Beta receptors do different things depending on where they are and which type of beta receptors they are. There are beta1 and beta2 receptors. Beta1 receptors are mainly in the heart and beta2 receptors are mainly in the lungs. When a beta blocker that can't tell the difference between a beta1 or beta2 is used, it not only blocks the beta1 in the heart which can lower blood pressure by decreasing the force of the heart's contractions but it also blocks the beta2 in the lungs which increases the difficulty of moving air in the airways. Lowering blood pressure can be good for you but making it harder to breathe at the same time can be bad for you.

If you must use a beta blocker, make sure your doctor orders a beta blocker that can tell the difference between the beta1 and beta2. The beta blockers that can tell the difference between beta receptors are called cardioselective beta blockers. That means the beta blocker 'selects' only the 'cardio' (heart) receptors. If you have a heart problem and you're prescribed a beta blocker to help your heart, a cardioselective beta blocker will block only the beta1 receptors and leave the beta2 receptors (in your lungs) alone.

A short list of cardioselective beta blockers include acebutolol, atenolol, bisoprolol, esmolol, and metoprolol. These medicines will treat your heart problem without adding to your breathing problem. Check with your doctor and be sure that he/she understands that taking a beta blocker that can't tell the difference between a beta1 or beta2 receptor could be a problem for you. Remember to avoid all beta blockers that block both beta1 and beta2 receptors because your easy breathing depends on beta2 receptors *not being blocked*.

ACE Inhibitors

Angiotensin-converting enzyme (ACE) has a very useful function in the body. Its ultimate job is to increase your blood pressure by any means possible.

An increased blood pressure can be good sometimes. Imagine getting a really bad cut and your blood is pouring out. As the blood runs out, the blood pressure falls (the way a water hose acts when there is a hole in the water hose). You need to have pressure to get the blood to all parts of the body like the brain and other important organs. In cases like this, you want your pressure to stay up. The ACE works hard to get your pressure up for you.

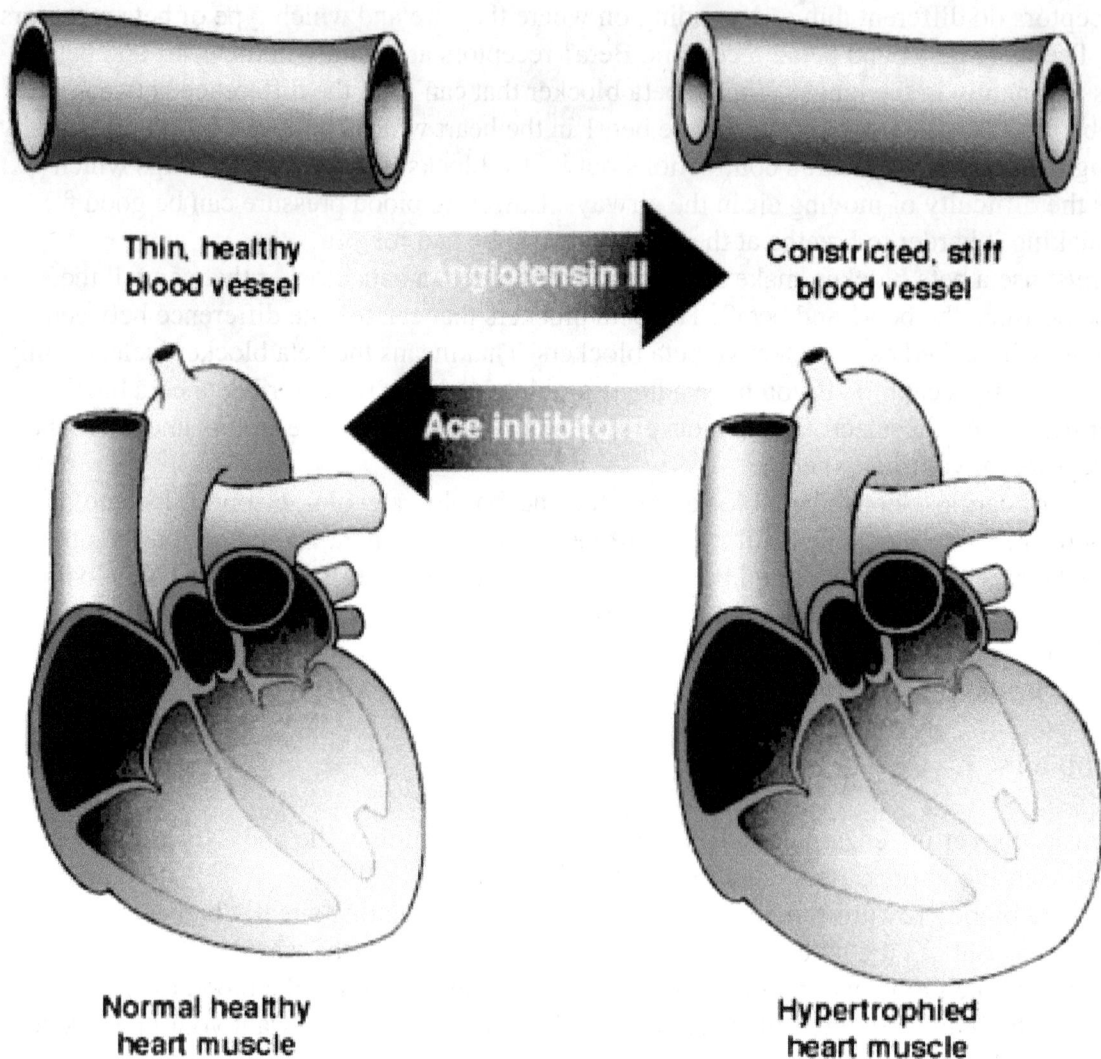

Thin, healthy
blood vessel

Angiotensin II

Ace inhibitors

Constricted, stiff
blood vessel

Normal healthy
heart muscle

Hypertrophied
heart muscle

There are also times when you want your pressure to be lower. Most of the time you'll rather your pressure to be lower than higher because higher pressures are not good for the blood vessels. Also, if your heart is ill, higher pressures increases the work your heart has to do and finally wears it out completely. So most of the time you'd rather have lower blood pressure.

To 'inhibit' means to hinder, restrain or prevent. For example: The cold inhibits plant growth. An ACE inhibitor prevents the angiotensin-converting enzyme from doing its job. What is the job of the angiotensin-converting enzyme? The enzyme is a coach that has been hired by the body to train angiotensin1 to be the super bad, really effective angiotensin2. The ACE inhibitor just kidnaps the coach, ties him up and throws him in the closet and sits on him. Now angiotensin1 never gets the training to become angiotensin2 and angiotensin1 is horrible at raising blood pressure.

There is a little trouble with the inhibitor. An ACE inhibitor can make you cough. One of the side effects of the ACE inhibitor is that it makes you cough and coughing can bring on an asthma attack. Among the list of ACE inhibitors are benazepril (Lotensin), captopril (Capoten), and lisinopril (Prinivil). If you're on either of these medicines or any other medicine ending in the letters P-R-I-L and if the medicine is making you cough a lot, ask your doctor to find a different medicine that does the same thing for you but doesn't make you cough.

Fortunately angiotensin receptor blockers (ARB) are medicines that lower blood pressure but don't cause coughing. Among the list of ARBs are candesartan (Atacand), valsartan (Diovan), and losartan (Cozaar). These medicines have their own side effects but causing you to cough excessively isn't one of them. Since coughing can start up an attack from the airway irritation that happens when you cough, you don't want to be coughing excessively if you can help it.

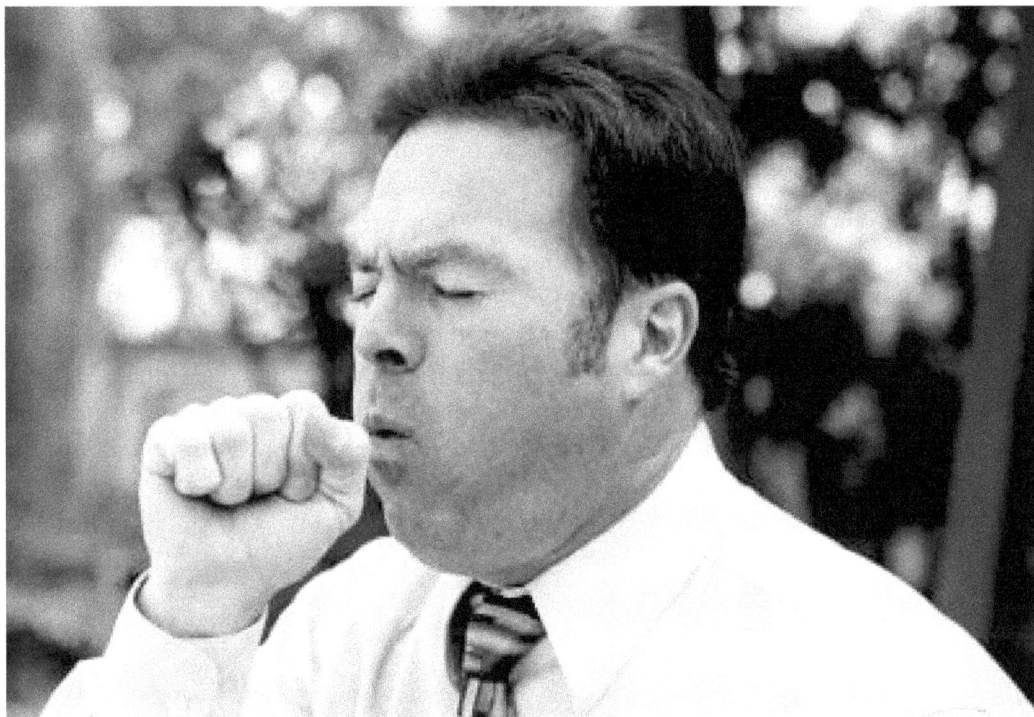

NSAIDs

Aspirin and other **N**on-**s**teroidal **a**nti-**i**nflammatory **d**rugs or NSAIDs are often used to treat inflammation. These medicines are now known to be harmful to as many as one in five adult asthmatics. Harmful in that aspirin can cause asthma attacks.

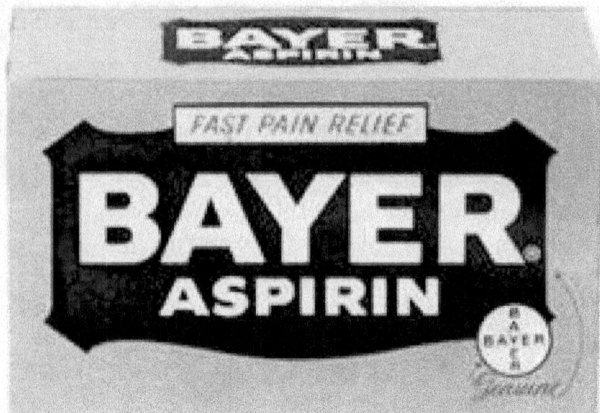

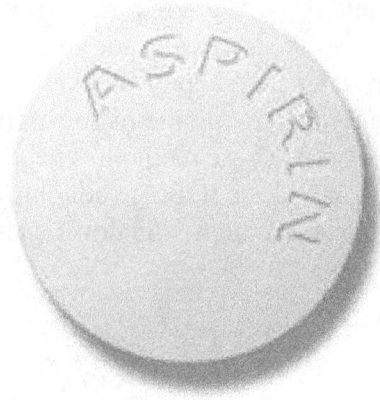

One in five adults and one in 20 children could be faced with bronchoconstriction and difficulty breathing after taking an aspirin.

If you become aware that you sometimes have trouble breathing after taking an aspirin, make sure that you tell your doctor. There are other medicines that do the same thing as aspirin but with a much less likelihood that you'll have an asthma attack afterwards.

The condition is called aspirin-induced asthma and it is more common to those in whom asthma is most severe. Older asthmatics are more likely to be subject to aspirin-induced asthma (AIA) also. Working with an allergy specialist could help you to reduce your sensitivity to aspirin if you must have aspirin. If your allergist and you are able to reduce your sensitivity, you must continue to take aspirin daily to maintain that.

Some alternative medicines to aspirin are acetaminophen (Tylenol) and the COX-2 inhibitor celecoxib.

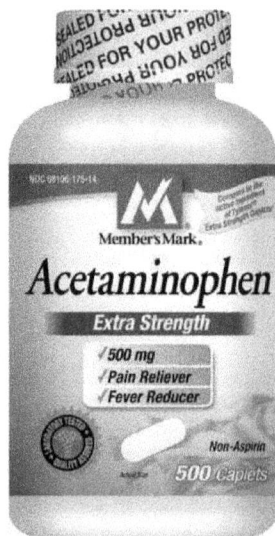

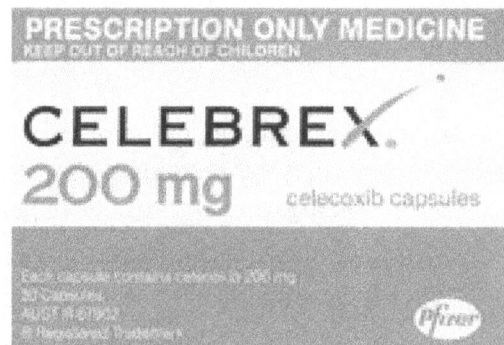

If you have another condition that require an anti-inflammatory, you'd be at less risk of worsening your breathing with these other options. Of course you should check with your doctor to make sure that these alternative medicines are OK for you and that they would be effective in the treatment for which aspirin was prescribed.

Sulfites

Sulfites are used as a food and beverage preservative. The Expert Panel recommends if you discover that your asthma flares up after you've eaten certain foods, it might be that you are allergic to sulfites and that you should avoid that food.

Sulfites are used to preserve dried fruits and potato products. Sulfites are also added to wine to arrest fermentation and to prevent spoilage. Generally, sweet wines contain more sulfites than dry wines and some sweet white wines contain more sulfites than red wines. In the US, if a wine was bottled after 1987 and has more than 10 parts per million of sulfites, a label must tell you so.

In 1986 the Food and Drug Administration banned the addition of sulfites to fruits and vegetables that would be eaten raw. You still have to be on the lookout for shrimp which sometimes have sulfites added to it on fishing boats and some beers still have sulfites added. Overall, the food landscape is somewhat safer but you still must be careful to avoid a possible fatal asthma attack due to your eating or drinking sulfites.

How to Recognize and Treat Worsening Asthma

How to recognize when your asthma is starting to give you trouble and what to do about it is the whole reason for this book. By this point, you've seen the important differences between your quick-relief and controller medicines. You've read what pulmonary functions are all about and you understand the importance of being in the know about your pulmonary functions. You know what triggers are and you've been given some ways to avoid some of them. You've been introduced to some of the tools and devices to use when you take different breathing medicines. You've even been warned away from some medicines and substances which could cause your asthma to flare up.

All of this information is leading to this: How to know when your asthma is getting bad and what are you supposed to do about it.

The Expert Panel met for the fourth time in 2007 with recommendations for asthma management and treatment. They provided direction on what to look for whether you are caring for an infant or child with asthma, an adolescent with asthma or an adult with asthma.

The Panel separated into three simple categories the information which will guide you to good decision making in what to do when trying to manage your asthma. Those categories are Well Controlled Asthma, Not Well Controlled Asthma, and Very Poorly Controlled Asthma. Which category includes your asthma condition is first decided by how old you are. Then by two groups of components which determine how severe your asthma is (current impairment) and how likely it is that you'll have future attacks (future risks).

The Expert Panel divided ages into three groups: Zero to four years, five to eleven years and twelve years and older. The things that would mark you as Well Controlled are a little different depending on if you're a baby or an adult. The symptoms and other signs which tell you what your asthma is doing are more important in one age group than in another. The same signs are considered but the seriousness of each sign is weighted a little differently depending on age.

Let's now look at the different age groups and see what conditions makes each Well Controlled, Not Well Controlled, and Very Poorly Controlled.

Zero to Four Years

(Well Controlled)

When your asthma is well controlled, the severity of your asthma is less and the chance of you having a huge flare-up is less. The same things that are looked at to see how well an adult's asthma is doing are the same things looked at to see how a baby's asthma is doing. Everything except for pulmonary function tests since babies up to four years old can't really do pulmonary functions. The other components are *symptoms, nighttime awakenings, interference with normal activity, and use of quick-relief medicines for symptom control*.

A child whose asthma is well controlled by this standard of the Expert Panel has wheezing or difficulty breathing less often than two days a week. Even when there is an episode of wheezing, it usually would happen only once that day.

Waking up at night because of trouble breathing is a sign that asthma is not perfectly controlled. However, we know that it is impossible to perfectly control all symptoms of asthma. If a child wakes up at night no more than once a month because of trouble breathing, this is considered acceptable. This child's condition would still be considered well controlled.

A child cannot have *any* interference with his or her normal activity and still be considered to have well controlled asthma. If a child of three, for example, can't run and play in the usual way without wanting to rest more than is common for that child, the child's asthma is not considered to be well controlled.

How often your child needs quick-relief medicines is another way to see how well controlled is the asthma. Usually this SABA (acting beta agonist) use will follow very closely with the symptoms. For a baby up to four years old, using quick-relief medicines two or fewer days per week is considered good. This would be considered well controlled asthma.

If your child has well controlled asthma, he or she shouldn't have a really bad flare up that causes your doctor to order oral steroids. Oral steroids are the steroids that are used when asthma is out of control and needs to be quickly brought back into control. A short course of oral systemic steroids over a period of a couple of weeks can reduce inflammation and regain normal airway function. If your child hasn't needed a little oral systemic steroid help no more than once in a year, the child's asthma is well controlled.

When your child's asthma is well controlled, you will not need to change the maintenance treatment routine you've been following. Simply use the quick-relief medicine when needed for wheezing and difficulty breathing and continue to use the inhaled steroid everyday if it has been prescribed.

There are a few signs you can look for to help you tell if the asthma is flaring up. Look for faster breathing especially when your baby is quiet, eating, or sleeping. Faster breathing often means trouble breathing. The faster the breathing, the more trouble the child is in.

Notice the nose of the child. If it is flaring (the nose holes are opening and closing noticeably), this usually means that the child is having trouble breathing. The faster the nose holes are opening and closing, the more trouble the child is having.

Tracheal tugging is a medical expression that means the dimple in the center of the neck right between the collar bones is appearing and disappearing as the child breathes in and out. Deeper dimples mean deeper trouble. Tracheal tugging is a sure sign of trouble breathing.

Finally, if you look at the ribs of your baby, if the skin between the ribs are sucking in and out when the child breathes, this is a clear sign of trouble breathing. The deeper the ribs are being sucked in, the deeper the trouble the child is in.

If your child has well controlled asthma, these signs of breathing trouble should not be often seen.

Zero to Four Years
(Not Well Controlled)

A child whose asthma is not well controlled will be noticed to have breathing trouble more often than a child whose asthma is well controlled.

The same measures of control (symptoms, nighttime awakenings, use of short acting beta agonists which is the same as quick-relief medicines, and big flare-ups requiring oral systemic corticosteroids) are considered.

A child from zero to four years old whose asthma is not well controlled will have symptoms of wheezing or other signs of difficulty breathing more often than two days weekly. The child might have several episodes during one or two days that week. You might notice fast breathing, nasal flaring, tracheal tugging, intercostal retractions (the ribs sucking in during breathing), excessive coughing, or you might hear wheezing. These will be noticeable and whether you see one sign or all the signs, any of them will tell you there is trouble. Your child's asthma is not well controlled.

Nighttime awakenings because of trouble breathing will happen more often. More than once a month of waking up with trouble breathing for a child in this age group will mean that his or her asthma is not well controlled.

Your child's asthma will interfere with his normal activities if his asthma is not well controlled. He will be less able to run and play with the same energy as his peers and friends. She might require more daytime naps because she gets tired more easily. Not well controlled asthma will show itself in the everyday activities of your child.

Symptoms that occur more often mean more use of quick-relief medicines. If your child is using albuterol or other quick-relief medicine more than two days a week, your child's asthma is not well controlled. This is why your doctor asks how long does your quick-relief inhaler last. To try to tell if the asthma you're treating is well controlled or not.

When asthma is not well controlled, there will likely be more visits to the emergency department. Here, doctors will attempt to get quick control of the asthma by giving an oral systemic corticosteroid. If this has happened two to three times in a year, your child's asthma is not well controlled.

It is very important that you recognize when your child has asthma that is not well controlled. Your actions will be aimed at managing the symptoms you see based on these descriptions of 'not well controlled' asthma.

Your short acting beta agonist (SABA) prescription will usually come with a recommended range of puffs to treat asthma symptoms. You should follow the direction of your action plan if you have one. The symptoms of a 'not well controlled' asthma would probably match well with the *yellow zone* of an action plan. You should then follow the medical directions for that zone. If you don't have a plan, follow the upper range of puffs to attempt to gain control of the asthma. For example, if the range allows 2-4 puffs when needed, try four puffs when you've noticed your child having continued trouble. Putting the upper range of puffs on a schedule like 'every four hours' or 'every three hours' for a couple of days might return your child to his or her 'normal.'

If you have a prescription for oral steroids, giving those as prescribed for usually 3-10 days will also help to get control of asthma that is 'not well controlled.'

It would certainly be smart to contact your doctor to tell him or her of your child's condition. Depending on your child's history, you might be asked to come to the hospital or urgent care clinic right away.

Zero to Four Years
(Very Poorly Controlled)

When a child's asthma is very poorly controlled, every measure of asthma severity is increased. Asthma symptoms will occur more often. More short acting beta agonists will be used for breathing relief. Asthma will interfere in a bigger way on everyday living and it will happen more often. Very poorly controlled asthma will result in more emergency department visits and more steroid prescriptions. Every sign that measures how bad the asthma is will be more noticeable.

Symptoms will go on throughout the day. The child will likely wake up with wheezing and go to bed with wheezing. There will be few moments which will find your child symptom free when his asthma is very poorly controlled.

If you are doing all you can do to control his asthma, nothing more can be done and it is what it is. However, if you haven't attempted to rid your home environment of possible allergens, if you haven't kept regular appointments with your doctor, if you haven't explored what allergy specialists might be able to offer, if you haven't used inhaled steroids consistently as prescribed and taken care to keep current with prescriptions, there might be a number of things that you could be doing to improve asthma control.

There will be extreme limitation on normal daily activities if a child in this age group has asthma that is very poorly controlled. These are the children who will be deeply affected by every lung irritant that is inhaled. Unable to even play in the park because of likely exposure to plant allergens that would make very poorly controlled asthma even worse. Those with very poorly controlled asthma will find even light exertion a problem.

With symptoms happening throughout the day, quick-relief medicines will be used several times a day to try to handle those symptoms. You would need to have SABAs (short acting beta agonists) in the car, in the house, at school or daycare, and the babysitters. You can't take the chance of your child needing his relief medicine and not having it because things could get really bad fast.

Emergency department visits would become fairly routine to you. Very poorly controlled asthma will require more than three visits a year to the ED and each visit would likely call for an oral steroid prescription. This places your child in that group of asthmatics who are at a higher risk of asthma related death.

If your child has very poorly controlled asthma, you should seek medical attention at the first sign of trouble. Since there will normally be a low level of control you should have phone numbers of your doctor, emergency departments, ambulance service, and urgent care centers always at the ready. You should have your asthma action plan memorized and know what symptoms show a dip in control. You'd be looking for an increase in how fast the child breathes, any bluish coloration of lips, wheezing, coughing or any signs of increased breathing distress.

To treat a child whose very poorly controlled asthma is worsening, you should go immediately to the emergency department. Until you get there you could give SABA and any oral steroid if you have any but you shouldn't delay. Very poorly controlled asthma that has become worse has turned into a life and death situation. This child will need medicines and monitoring equipment that you wouldn't have at home so getting to a medical facility will be your top priority.

**Five to Eleven Years
(Well Controlled)**

Children in this age group have larger airways than the younger group. They are bigger children so generally their airways can handle more stress than the smaller children. These differences don't become noticeable until their asthma is 'not well controlled' and 'very poorly controlled.' Most of the components which measure asthma control in the 'well controlled' category of asthma control are the same for the zero to four years and the five to eleven years age groups. The only difference is that by the age of five years old, pulmonary functions can be tested.

Remember that pulmonary functions for asthmatics measure how easily or hard it is to blow air out of the lungs. When it is easier to blow air out, more can be blown out in less time. The Forced Expired Volume (FEV) in 1 second is a measure of that ease. Usually a visit to the pulmonary functions lab is needed to do an FEV1. A peak flow can be done at home and it is also a measure of the ease or difficulty of blowing air out of the lungs. Either of these tests are useful measures of how well controlled your child's asthma is.

An FEV1 of more than 80% tells you that your child's asthma is well controlled. This means that more than eighty percent of the air in your child's lungs can be blown out in 1 second. This also says that there is not much obstruction in the airway and your child can breathe very easily. A peak flow reading of more than 80% of what is normal for your child is good. Your child is at least eighty percent of what is predicted for children his age and size. The peak flow also says that your child is able to blow at least eighty percent of what he is normally able to blow. He's more than eighty percent as good as he ever is at getting air out of his lungs.

Another PFT (pulmonary function test) measure is the FEV1/FVC ratio. The FVC is the Forced Vital Capacity. The total amount of air that can be forcibly blown out of your lungs. This is a yardstick that the Expert Panel also felt to be very useful in measuring how well controlled your asthma is. The more air that can be blown out in 1 second, the higher the ratio. The higher the ratio, the more well controlled is your asthma. A ratio of greater than 80% points to asthma that is well controlled. A child in this age group who has 'well controlled' asthma would have an FEV1 and an FEV1/FVC of more than 80%.

Treatment of your child's asthma when it is in this 'well controlled' category is easy. Just continue doing what your doctor has instructed you to do. Give the inhaled steroid consistently every day if it has been prescribed. Give the quick-relief medicine when needed. Be alert for changes in symptoms like how fast your child is breathing, increasing restlessness, or a slow down in playing for example.

**Five to Eleven Years
(Not Well Controlled)**

A child in this age group would have very similar experiences as the children in the zero to four age group. Symptoms of difficulty breathing, wheezing, excessive coughing and other signs of trouble breathing would happen just about as often as in the younger age group--more than two days a week or several times on any given day.

Use of quick-relief medicine would pick up too as you try to control the more frequent symptoms. More than two days weekly or several times on any given day you'll have to give treatments to a child in the 'not well controlled' category.

Interruptions in nighttime sleep would happen more often too as the child is awakened with coughing, wheezing and chest tightness.

Interference with your child's daily activities would be noticeable. You might notice that he or she doesn't ask to go bike riding as often. You might notice that he gets tired more easily if he is active or that he's harder to budge from his room to go outside to be active. There will definitely be some limitation on your child's activity levels in this 'not well controlled' category.

In this age group you'll be able to measure how well the lung is functioning. A pulmonary function test (PFT) would allow you to measure an FEV1 and an FEV1/FVC. If you have a peak flow meter you'll be able to use this tool to get an idea of your child's lung function. These tests provide numbers that can clearly show when asthma is not being well controlled.

An FEV1 in a child with 'not well controlled' asthma would be between sixty and eighty percent. These numbers are clearly different now that the asthma is 'not well controlled.' The ratio of the FEV1/FVC would also drop noticeably from more than 80 percent in well controlled asthma to between seventy-five and eighty percent. Peak flows on the peak flow meter would match what the FEV1 is and fall between 60 and 80 percent.

Keeping a peak flow meter around to measure your child's ease of blowing out air is a great way to see how well controlled or not well controlled her asthma is. Peak flow meters are convenient to have since they don't require appointments to the pulmonary function lab but they still give useful numbers to help you keep up with your child's asthma.

If your child's asthma is 'not well controlled,' the risk is increased that he'll have to be rushed to the emergency department for breathing trouble. You can expect that you'll have to rush him to the emergency department two or more times a year to get treatment for his asthma. This will usually involve a short course of oral steroids to help regain control. It is the oral systemic corticosteroids that bring the most risk of steroid side effects, though these risks are very small.

When your child's asthma is not well controlled, you should try to improve his breathing when you notice any signs of trouble. An action plan would come in very useful at times like these since the asthma action plan can function as the clear thinking caregiver since you'll probably be nervous and not at your best.

First give the quick-relief medicine, usually albuterol but it could be Xopenex or Maxair. Give what you usually give to bring relief. Wait twenty minutes for results. If you don't see noticeable improvement, give the upper limit of the dose range which is usually a little more than what you usually give. If this seems to work and the signs of distress (wheezing, coughing, complaints of chest tightness) goes away, give the quick-relief medicine on a schedule for a couple of days. Three to four puffs (depending on the age and size of your child) every four hours if it's albuterol (it might be a little different if it's another medicine. Check with your doctor or pharmacist). Follow this schedule of regular quick-relief medicine for a couple of days. Continue with the inhaled steroids if you have them. Call your doctor to keep him or her informed of your child's condition. You might need to make an appointment to get up to date information on how well controlled you child's asthma is now.

If you've given the albuterol or other quick-relief medicine but don't see any improvement after the second treatment, make plans to get to a medical facility. You can continue with the treatments even as you make your way to the emergency department. If your child seem to be getting worse, call an ambulance. An ambulance will likely have medicines that you don't have and they will also be able to monitor other measures of your child's condition that you don't have equipment to monitor.

The hardest part of treating your child's asthma when it has become 'not well controlled' is being aware that the asthma condition has changed. Always be alert for change especially after exposure to possible or known triggers. Once you've recognized that the asthma condition has changed, acting on the knowledge right away is important. Don't wait until morning to treat the asthma if you discover the change at night. Change in your child's condition can be fast moving and treating the asthma now rather than later is the right thing to do.

Five to Eleven Years
(Very Poorly Controlled)

Very poorly controlled asthma threatens your child's life. If you're doing all that you can do but the asthma is still out of control, you must consider several of the following things:

1. Is your living environment causing some of this trouble? Is your child exposed to things he or she is allergic to like smoke or animal dander? Removing those allergens and irritants from the home could help a great deal in controlling your child's asthma.

2. Does your child have some other health condition that is complicating his asthma like GERD (gastroesophageal reflux disease) or rhinitis?

3. Is your child using medicines that are known to work against asthmatics like beta blockers? Are foods containing sulfites being eaten?

These are a few of the questions that you must ask to effectively manage asthma that is 'very poorly controlled.'

Very poorly controlled asthma will leaving your child symptomatic most of the time. Throughout the day she'll complain of difficulty breathing or she'll be coughing or wheezing. She won't be much better off at night. She'll awake with trouble breathing two or more times a week. Not getting a good night's sleep could interfere with her alertness in school so that her grades could suffer.

She'll go through canisters of albuterol or other quick-relief medicines quickly since you'll be using it several times a day to control her symptoms. Using these short acting beta agonists too often can, over time, cause these medicines to become less effective at relieving distress.

She'll have to deal with extreme limitation on her daily activities. It is unlikely that she'll be able to play any kind of team sport or even dance or tennis since her breathing trouble would be so constant. All but the mildest exertions would probably cause attacks so everything except the necessary activities would be cut out.

Pulmonary functions would be low even when she's at her best if her asthma is very poorly controlled. You'd see FEV1 at less than 60%. That means she'd be able to blow only sixty percent of her air out in 1 second. That's very bad. Her FEV1/FVC ratio would be less than seventy-five percent. Peak flows would also be less than sixty percent. That means if she can blow 350 on her flow meter when she's doing very good, she'd blow less than 210 when her asthma is very poorly controlled.

You can expect that she'll need a boost of oral systemic steroids two or more times each year to help gain control of her asthma.

Very poorly controlled asthma puts your child at risk of side effects from the steroids, life threatening flare-ups and gradual reshaping of airways.

Treatment of asthma that is very poorly controlled is all about recognizing change. Faster breathing or noticeable wheezing when you hadn't noticed it before says that asthma is changing for the worse. Sitting with shoulders raised, propped on hands like a tripod is a sign of asthma that is out of control. Uncontrollable coughing that seems endless is a mark of extreme distress requiring immediate action. Complaints of chest tightness or inability to breathe are cries for help and a sign that you should get ready to go to the hospital or call an ambulance. If you notice that peak flows are down or symptoms are happening more often, get to the hospital right away. If very poorly controlled asthma is your child's normal, she would not be able to withstand even a small drop in her condition before her situation would become very serious.

You should always have quick-relief medicine available everywhere your child is expected to be; school, car, home, and family members' homes. Keep all prescriptions current and filled. Never allow yourself to run out of any of them for any reason. Give all prescribed medicines consistently. Keep your action plan where you can find it and make sure you understand everything on it.

If you notice that you child's asthma is changing for the worse, give quick-relief medicines right away to try to help your child breathe. You might have steroids at home for worsening asthma. If you do, give that amount that your doctor says is the right amount for your child's age and weight. Then go immediately to the emergency department. Delay is not what you want to do if your child has very poorly controlled asthma.

Twelve Years Old to Adult
(Well Controlled)

Well controlled asthma is to older children and adults as it is to babies and younger children. You see fewer symptoms of asthma such as wheezing and chest tightness or coughing. You are less often awakened at night by breathing trouble. You'd use your quick-relief medicines less often to battle your symptoms which would be happening less often. Your daily activities would be less effected by your asthma condition and you'd be less likely to have to rush to an emergency department for treatment.

The only differences you'd notice between young children and twelve year olds and older are small differences between numbers. How many times per week you'd have nighttime awakenings, for example, before your asthma control changes categories from 'well controlled' to 'not well controlled.' This is just a little different from those numbers which define the age category of 'five to eleven years.' The reason is primarily because of the size of the asthmatics involved. Generally, bigger kids have bigger airways and can withstand a similar insult to the airway with a milder asthmatic response. An irritant that might close off a smaller airway might still leave a little breathing hole in a larger airway. This could be the difference between treating that condition yourself and rushing immediately to the nearest medical facility.

These measures of asthma control which have defined the previous two categories will be used again to define this last 'twelve years old to adult' category.

Symptoms of breathing difficulty such as wheezing, coughing excessively or complaints of chest tightness, would be seen on two or fewer days per week. If your asthma is in the 'well controlled' category you would have your sleep disrupted by trouble breathing no more than two times a month. With so little trouble, your days would go smoothly and you'd easily be able to forget that you even have asthma.

Your canisters of quick-relief medicine would last you longer since you'd be using SABAs or short acting beta agonists less often to control your symptoms. You'd need to use your quick-relief medicines no more than two days a week.

Your daily activities would be easier for you because your asthma wouldn't interfere. Your asthma would be so well controlled that you could take the stairs as easily as you could take the elevator. If your job required you to move around on your feet much of the day, you could probably do that without a problem.

If your asthma is well controlled, your peak flow and pulmonary function results would show this through higher numbers (peak flow) and higher percentages (FEV1). Your forced expired volume in 1 second would be more than eighty percent of what is normal for you and others like you (others of similar age, gender, and height according to prediction charts). Your peak flow would read that you're blowing out more than 80% of what you blow out when you're at your best.

You'd have no more that one big flare-up a year that would cause you to have to take oral systemic corticosteroids. Your asthma is well controlled so you're doing just fine.

Treatment of a little flare-up would be to simply take the usual dose of your quick-relief medicine. Your condition would be easy to manage if your asthma is already well controlled. If you've been prescribed daily inhaled steroids, you should be taking your medicine everyday as prescribed. Consistently taking your medicines as the doctor has ordered is most of the reason your asthma is well controlled and easy to manage. Be watchful of any changes in how often your symptoms occur or how bad they might be and be prepared to increase your dose of quick-relief medicine accordingly.

Even well controlled asthma can sometimes have a serious flare-up so remember to avoid your triggers and to keep your quick-relief medicines on hand.

Twelve Years Old to Adult
(Not Well Controlled)

Asthma that is not well controlled in this age category is easy to recognize. The measures of control which were used to describe the other age categories and levels of control are used again to describe 'not well controlled' asthma in this age category.

Symptoms would be unavoidable. Wheezes, chest tightness, excessive coughing or other signs of distress would happen more than two days a week. This means that you would often have trouble with your asthma.

You would use more quick-relief medicine to handle your more frequent symptoms. Your symptoms would be happening more than two days a week and you'd be using your medicine more than two days a week. You'd go through your inhalers more quickly since you'd be using the SABAs more often.

From once to three times a week you'd wake up at night with trouble breathing. Wheezing, coughing, chest tightness or some other symptom of your breathing distress would interrupt your night's rest every other day on average.

Your normal activity would definitely be interfered with by your asthma. Your 'not well controlled' asthma would decide many things for you like where you park when you go shopping. You wouldn't want to have to walk too far with that load of groceries. It would decide whether you catch an elevator or take the stairs. You could be on the verge of an attack by the time you'd reached your destination if you had to climb a few flights of stairs to get there. It would even decide whether you exercise, how much exercise and what type of exercise you do.

If you're in school and hoped to participate in team sports, you could probably forget that. 'Not well controlled' asthma would be too unstable and would need to much medicine and support to allow you to join a sports team. Having 'not well controlled asthma' would leave you always at risk for a serious attack at any time.

Your FEV1 and peak flow would be between sixty and eighty percent. Saying this another way, if your asthma is not well controlled you would be able to breathe only 60 to 80% as well as you need to.

You would be at increased risk of having a serious, life threatening asthma attack. It is likely that you would need to go to the emergency department for a short course of steroids to help turn your worsening asthma around. You could expect to need at least two or more oral steroid prescriptions per year if your asthma is not well controlled.

Treatment of 'not well controlled' asthma would involve using your quick-relief medicine when you discover that your asthma is worsening.

If you notice that you're getting tired more easily than you usually do, that you're wheezing more, or if you can feel your chest tightening, use your quick-relief inhaler. You should give yourself a couple more puffs than you do ordinarily when you feel a little short of breath. Put yourself on a schedule for quick-relief puffs every 4-6 hrs for a couple of days to try to improve your breathing. If you notice that you're feeling better and you feel like your asthma is improving, continue the schedule for a couple of days. Take some oral steroids if they've been prescribed to you and take the amount your doctor has said is the right amount for you to take. If you feel like it isn't working, call your doctor and go to a health care facility for professional help. Never try to just 'gut it out' or push through it. An asthma attack is a medical emergency.

You should have an asthma action plan to tell you what you should do at times when your asthma is not doing well. You should make sure that you understand your plan. At times when your distress is high, you might not be able to think as clearly as you normally do. It would be helpful if you have an asthma action plan to do the thinking for you.

Keep all medicines mentioned in your plan available to you. Don't allow yourself to run out of them. Keep them refilled. When you're facing a breathing emergency, you don't want to reach for your 'quick-relief' and discover that there'll be no relief because you've run out of medicine.

Twelve Years Old to Adult
(Very Poorly Controlled)

Very poorly controlled asthma is trouble in any age category. It could be the result of constant exposure to triggers or failing to take medicines as prescribed. It could also simply be the result of asthma that is just very difficult to control.

If you have been prescribed steroid inhalers you should take them. Your asthma will only get worse and harder to manage if you don't. If you've identified triggers that cause your asthma to flare up, you should carefully avoid those triggers or your asthma will only be more bothersome to you. You should have your pulmonary functions checked routinely, at least once or twice a year or whenever you have a serious flare-up to always know the condition of your asthma. A peak flowmeter is very appropriate for 'very poorly controlled' asthma.

Very poorly controlled asthma requires more types of medicines to keep it under control. You might have immunomodulators, long acting beta agonists, even oral steroids in medium to large doses to keep some control over your asthma. You should take these medicines as the doctor has prescribed. The alternative is asthma that is not controlled and that is simply not a choice to consider.

As in the other age categories, the same measures of asthma control are used to understand how well controlled your asthma is.

Symptoms of trouble breathing, chest tightness, excessive coughing or wheezing will be present throughout the day. If not these symptoms then there will be some other symptoms of trouble breathing.

Nighttime awakenings due to trouble breathing will be almost every night. It will be a rare night that you're not awakened with coughing or other sign of trouble breathing. Be sure to check with your doctor to make sure you aren't dealing with something else and asthma too. For example obesity can cause you to wake up at night if your breathing is being blocked by soft tissue in your neck. You could also be dealing with GERD (gastroesophageal reflux disease) which could wake you up in the middle of the night with breathing discomfort.

Several times daily you'll have to reach for your inhaler to get relief from your asthma symptoms. You'll use your quick-relief medicine often.

Your everyday activities will be decided by how bad your asthma is. There will be constant interference from your 'very poorly controlled' asthma. Forget about engaging in sports or exercise. You would have too little control over your asthma to permit chasing a ball or jogging. Your focus will be on simply getting along through the day with as little disruption as possible to your daily life. Your very poorly controlled asthma would be in control of you.

You would be well known at your local emergency department where you would have visited at least two or more times a year for treatment. At those times, oral steroids would have been given to try to take control of your asthma. You would be at serious risk of life threatening attacks when your asthma is very poorly controlled.

When you have asthma this poorly controlled, it is very hard to treat at home. You can only give yourself quick-relief medicine as you make your way to a medical facility. You might consider calling an ambulance to come for you since, if things should take a turn for the worse, they would have some life saving equipment that you wouldn't have.

The best way to effectively treat very poorly controlled asthma is to always be aware of what condition your asthma is in. Treat it before it gets really bad. If you see that your quick-relief inhalers are less effective than they usually are, see your doctor. Your condition will likely get worse before it gets better. When you seem more short of breath than you usually are, see your doctor. Your asthma is most likely getting worse and your medicines might need adjusting. When the time of the year when you see most of your asthma trouble gets near, see your doctor. You might be able to control how bad your asthma gets. Being constantly aware of your asthma condition will help to manage it better.

Additional Resources

This book is a great source of information about asthma. I've included a list of additional sources that will tell you all you could want to know about asthma. These resources were taken directly from the Expert Panel's third report on asthma and they include phone numbers and websites. One or more of these organizations will be able to answer any of your questions that you might have after reading this book.

Allergy & Asthma Network Mothers of Asthmatics
2751 Prosperity Avenue, Suite 150
Fairfax, VA 22030
1–800–878–4403
1–703–641–9595
www.breatherville.org

American Academy of Allergy, Asthma and Immunology
555 East Wells Street, Suite 100
Milwaukee, WI 53202-3823
1–414–272–6071
www.aaaai.org

American Association For Respiratory Care
9125 North MacArthur Boulevard, Suite 100
Irving, TX 75063
1–972–243–2272
www.aarc.org

American College of Allergy, Asthma, and Immunology
85 West Algonquin Road 1–847–427–1200
Suite 550
Arlington Heights, IL 60005
1–800–842–7777
www.Acaai.Org

American Lung Association
61 Broadway
New York, NY 10006
1–800–586–4872
www.lungusa.org

Association of Asthma Educators
1215 Anthony Avenue
Columbia, SC 29201
1–888–988–7747
www.asthmaeducators.org

Asthma and Allergy Foundation of America
1233 20th Street, NW., Suite 402
Washington, DC 20036
1–800–727–8462
www.aafa.org

Centers for Disease Control and Prevention
1600 Clifton Road
Atlanta, GA 30333
1–800–311–3435

Food Allergy & Anaphylaxis Network
11781 Lee Jackson Highway, Suite 160
Fairfax, VA 22033
1–800–929–4040
www.foodallergy.org

National Heart, Lung, and Blood Institute Information Center
P.O. Box 30105
Bethesda, MD 20824-0105
1–301–592–8573
www.nhlbi.nih.gov

National Jewish Medical and Research Center (Lung Line)
1400 Jackson Street
Denver, CO 80206
1–800–222–Lung
www.njc.org

U.S. Environmental Protection Agency
National Center for Environmental Publications
P.O. Box 42419
Cincinnati, OH 45242-0419
1–800–490–9198
www.airnow.gov

Asthma Medicine Prices
Taken from CanadaDrugs.com except as listed

   The Food and Drug Administration has phased out or will soon phase out the following medicines so these are not listed on this price list: Aerobid (6/30/11), Alupent (6/14/10), Azmacort (12/31/10), Tilade (6/14/10), Intal (12/31/10), Maxair (12/31/13)and Combivent (12/31/13). Discontinuance is due to US obligations under the Montreal Protocol related to depletion of the ozone layer.

Pulmicort (generic equivalent) 0.5mg/2ml nebule   20 nebules for $43.33
Asmanex 200 mcg 60 doses for $99.42
Flovent 44 mcg 120 dose for $31.40
Flovent 110 mcg 120 dose for $37.73
Flovent 220 mcg 120 dose for $68.60
Qvar 50 mcg 200 dose for $40.50
Qvar 100 mcg 200 dose for $96.79
Alvesco 80 mcg 120 dose for $103.68
Alvesco 160 mcg 120 dose for $120.80

Xolair 150mg: $541 (for 2 weeks), $1,082 (for 4 weeks) *not found at CanadaDrugs.com*
        375mg: $1,353 (for 2 weeks), $2,706 (for 4 weeks)

Singulair 10mg 28 tablets for $59.30
Singulair Chewables 5mg 28 tablets for $58.20
Singulair granules 4mg 28 packet for $69.40

Zyflo (northdrugstore.com) 600mg 120 tablets for $1,191.00. Generic zileuton 600mg 100 tablets for $325.00

Serevent Diskus 50mcg 60 dose $66.29
Serevent Inhaler 25mcg 120 dose $61.40
Foradil 12mcg 60 capsules $63.32, generic equivalent 12mcg 30 capsules $19.92

Quibron not found (Uniphyl 400mg is comparable alternate, 56 tablets $48.55)
Theo-24 200mg 30 capsules $32.41
Theo-Dur not found (Theophylline 300mg is comparable alternate, 100 tablets $30.60)

Dulera Inhaler 50mcg/5mcg 120 dose $187.20
Dulera Inhaler 100mcg/5mcg 120 dose $250.00
Dulera Inhaler 200mcg/5mcg 120 dose $240.00
Symbicort Turbuhaler 100mcg/6mcg 120 dose $95.25
Advair Diskus 100mcg/50mcg 60 dose $65.50
Advair Diskus 250mcg/50mcg 60 dose $71.32
Advair Diskus 500mcg/50mcg 60 dose $95.74

Salbutamol (same as Albuterol) 1mg/ml 20 nebule $20.31 (for nebulizers)
Salbutamol (same as Albuterol) 0.5mg/ml 20 nebule $19.20 (for nebulizers)

Salbutamol CFC Free Inhaler 100mcg (generic equivalent to Ventolin) 200 dose $15.60
Levalbuterol Inhaler 0.045mg (generic equivalent to Xopenex) 200 dose $32.60

Atrovent Inhaler 20mcg/ds 200 dose 43.81
Ipratropium Inhalation Solution 500mcg/2ml (generic Atrovent) 20 ampule $29.64

Prednisone 1mg 100 tablets $22.75
Prednisone 2.5mg 100 tablets $32.23
Pediapred Oral Liquid 5mg/5ml (equivalent to Prednisolone) 120ml $37.66

Peak Flowmeter Prices
by flow range, model number, retail outlet or manufacturer

Personal Best Peak Flowmeter   HDNHS756012   Low Range 50-360LPM
$18.57 by respironics/healthdyne

Tru-zone Peak Flowmeter   Invirc1198   Low and High range
 $12.94 by Invacare Corporation

Omron Peak Flowmeter   unbeatablesale.com $27.25

Standard Model Assess Peak Flowmeter   ebay.com $15.49

AsthmaMentor Peak Flowmeter   Low and High range   HS742-010 $21.91

Microlife Digital Peak Flow & FEV1 Meter drugstore.com $39.99

Mabis Peak Flowmeter   Walmart $24.99

Pocketpeak Peak Flowmeter   Low and High Range $17.77 to $39.88

Research Notes and References

The Expert Panel's third report was liberally referenced for this book. Over ninety-five percent of the material came from "Guidelines for the Diagnosis and Management of Asthma," the title of the Expert Panel's third report, commissioned by the National Asthma Education and Prevention Program. In those few instances where greater detail was needed about a particular subject, the sites referenced for that information is listed here.

AAAAI's contributors. (2012). *Mold Allergy.* Available: http://www.aaaai.org/conditions-and-treatments/allergies/mold-allergy.aspx. Last accessed 18th Nov 2012.

Bhargava,Hansa D. MD. (2012). Asthma and Sulfite Allergies.Available: http://www.webmd.com/asthma/asthma-and-sulfites-allergies. Last accessed 18th Nov 2012.

Conrad Stoppler,MD, M. (2012). Mold Exposure. Available: http://www.medicinenet.com/mold_exposure/article.htm. Last accessed 18th Nov 2012.

CDC contributors. (2012). Common Asthma Triggers. Available: http://www.cdc.gov/asthma/triggers.html. Last accessed 18th Nov 2012.

CDC contributors. (2012). Triggers Outdoors. Available: http://www.cdc.gov/asthma/triggers_outdoor.html. Last accessed 18th Nov 2012.

Editorial Board. (2005). Mold Allergy. Available: http://www.aafa.org/display.cfm?cont=58&id=8&sub=16. Last accessed 18th Nov 2012.

Editorial Group: Cochrane Airways Group.. (2008). Ciclesonide versus other inhaled steroids for chronic asthma in children and adults.Available: http://www.ncbi.nlm.nih.gov/pubmedhealth/PMH0014284/. Last accessed 17th Nov 2012.

ELIZABETH F. JUNIPER, PAUL M. O'BYRNE, PENELOPE J. FERRIE, DEREK R. KING and JEREMY N. ROBERTS. (2000). Measuring Asthma Control Clinic Questionnaire or Daily Diary? . Available: http://ajrccm.atsjournals.org/content/162/4/1330.full. Last accessed 18th Nov 2012.

Frea, R. (2010). Seven Classic Asthma Medicines to be Discontinued.Available: http://www.healthcentral.com/asthma/c/52325/109434/discontinued/. Last accessed 18th Nov 2012.

Genentech contributors. (2012). Who is Xolair for?. Available: http://www.xolair.com/xolair/index.html?cid=xol_we_F001114_P000517&c=MIXLAA8049&utm_source=google&utm_medium=cpc&utm_term=omalizumab&utm_campaign=2012%20Xolair%20Branded%20(Feb%2012)&gclid=CKnzse_ryLM. Last accessed 18th Nov 2012.

Healthy Learners Asthma Initiative. (2012). How to use the Maxair Autohaler. Available: http://www.health.state.mn.us/asthma/documents/maxairinstruc.pdf. Last accessed 18th Nov 2012.

iVillage Staff. (2012). Top Ten Indoor Plants. Available: http://www.ivillage.com/top-10-indoor-plants/7-a-258925. Last accessed 18th Nov 2012.

LIYA DAVYDOV, PHARM.D.. (2005). Omalizumab (Xolair) for Treatment of Asthma. Available: http://www.aafp.org/afp/2005/0115/p341.html. Last accessed 18th Nov 2012.

Mark Kosinski, Kathy Lampl and Sulabha Ramachandran Bradley Chipps, Robert S. Zeiger, Kevin Murphy, Michael Mellon, Michael Schatz,. (2011).Longitudinal Validation of the Test for Respiratory and Asthma Control in Kids in Pediatric Practices. Available: http://pediatrics.aappublications.org/content/early/2011/02/21/peds.2010-1465.full.pdf. Last accessed 18th Nov 2012.

Medicine.org.UK contributors. (2010). How to use your Turbohaler.Available: http://www.youtube.com/watch?v=sJdG-c6y84l. Last accessed 18th Nov 2012.

National Jewish Health contributors. (2009). Twisthaler. Available: http://www.youtube.com/watch?v=tyxAlhWaD0M. Last accessed 18th Nov 2012.

PubMed contributors. (2011). Gastroesophageal reflux disease.Available: http://www.ncbi.nlm.nih.gov/pubmedhealth/PMH0001311/. Last accessed 18th Nov 2012.

RAMP's contributors. (2009). Asthma Action Plans. Available: http://www.rampasthma.org/info-resources/asthma-action-plans/. Last accessed 18th Nov 2012.

Seidu,L MD. . (2012). Mold Allergy. Available: http://www.webmd.com/allergies/guide/mold-allergy. Last accessed 18th Nov 2012.

Tinkelman,D MD.. (2012). Using A Rotahaler. Available: http://www.nationaljewish.org/healthinfo/medications/lung-diseases/devices/dry-powder/rotahaler/. Last accessed 18th Nov 2012.

Tinkelman,D MD.. (2012). Using A Twisthaler. Available: http://www.nationaljewish.org/healthinfo/medications/lung-diseases/devices/dry-powder/twisthaler/. Last accessed 18th Nov 2012.

Weber, C MD. (2008). Can I Take Beta Blockers if I Have Asthma?.Available: http://highbloodpressure.about.com/od/treatmentmonitoring/f/asthma-beta.htm. Last accessed 18th Nov 2012.

WebMD contributors. (2012). Drugs and Medications- Maxair Autohaler Inhl. Available: http://www.webmd.com/drugs/drug-14096-Maxair+Autohaler+Inhl.aspx?drugid=14096&drugname=Maxair+Autohaler+Inhl. Last accessed 18th Nov 2012.

Wikipedia contributors. (2012). ACE inhibitor. Available: http://en.wikipedia.org/wiki/ACE_inhibitor. Last accessed 18th Nov 2012.

Wikipedia contributors. (2008). Aspirin-Induced Asthma. Available: http://en.wikipedia.org/wiki/Aspirin-induced_asthma. Last accessed 18th Nov 2012.

Wikipedia contributors. (2007). Laryngotracheal stenosis. Available: http://en.wikipedia.org/wiki/Laryngotracheal_stenosis. Last accessed 17th Nov 2012.

www.ingramcontent.com/pod-product-compliance
Lightning Source LLC
Chambersburg PA
CBHW080001280326
41935CB00013B/1716